D0084039

Course Notes and Workbook for Introduction to Sound

Acoustics for the Hearing and Speech Sciences

Third Edition

Singular Textbook Series
Series Editor: M.N. Hegde

Adult Neurogenic Language Disorders: Assessment and Treatment: An Ethnocentric Approach
By Joan C. Payne, Ph.D.

Anatomy and Physiology for Speech and Language
By J. Anthony Seikel, Ph.D., Douglas W. King, Ph.D., and David G. Drumright, B.S.

Applied Phonetics: The Sounds of American English (2nd ed.)
By Harold T. Edwards, Ph.D.

Applied Phonetics Workbook: A Systematic Approach to Phonetic Transcription (2nd ed.)
By Harold T. Edwards, Ph.D.

Applied Phonetics Instructor's Manual (2nd ed.)
By Harold T. Edwards, Ph.D.

Articulation and Phonological Disorders: A Book of Exercises (2nd ed.)
By Ken M. Bleile, Ph.D.

Assessment in Speech-Language Pathology, A Resource Manual (2nd ed.)
By Kenneth G. Shipley, Ph.D., and Julie McAfee, M.S.

Clinical Methods and Practicum in Speech-Language Pathology (2nd ed.)
By M.N. Hegde, Ph.D., and Deborah Davis, M.A.

Clinical Methods in Audiology
By Ben R. Kelly, Ph.D., Deborah Davis, M.S., and M.N. Hegde, Ph.D.

Clinical Speech and Voice Measurement: Laboratory Exercises
By Robert F. Orlikoff, Ph.D. and Ronald J. Baken, Ph.D.

Clinical Speech and Voice Measurement: Instructor's Manual
By Robert F. Orlikoff, Ph.D. and Ronald J. Baken, Ph.D.

A Coursebook on Aphasia (2nd ed.)
By M. N. Hegde, Ph.D.

A Coursebook on Language Disorders in Children
By M. N. Hegde, Ph.D.

A Coursebook on Scientific and Professional Writing in Speech-Language Pathology (2nd ed.)
By M. N. Hegde, Ph.D.

Diagnosis in Speech-Language Pathology
Edited by J. Bruce Tomblin, Ph.D., D. C. Spriestersbach, Ph.D., and Hughlett Morris, Ph.D.

Introduction to Clinical Research in Communication Disorders
By Mary Pannbacker, Ph.D., and Grace Middleton, Ed.D.

Introduction to Communication Disorders
Edited by Fred D. Minifie, Ph.D.

Student Workbook for Introduction to Communication Disorders
By Fred D. Minifie, Ph.D., with Carolyn R. Carter and Jason L. Smith

Instructor's Manual for Introduction to Communication Disorders
By Fred D. Minifie, Ph.D.

Introduction to Sound: Acoustics for the Hearing and Speech Sciences (3rd ed.)
By Charles E. Speaks, Ph.D.

Language and Deafness (2nd ed.)
By Peter V. Paul, Ph.D., and Stephen P. Quigley, Ph.D.

Study Guide for Language and Deafness (2nd ed.)
By Peter V. Paul, Ph.D.

Optimizing Theories and Experiments
By Randall R. Robey, Ph.D., and Martin C. Shultz, Ed.D.

Neuroscience of Communication (2nd ed.)
By Douglas B. Webster, Ph.D.

Professional Issuesin Communication Disorders
Edited by Rosemary Lubinski, Ed.D., and Carol Frattali, Ph.D.

The Acoustic Analysis of Speech
By Ray D. Kent, Ph.D., and Charles Read, Ph.D.

Also available:

A Singular Manual of Textbook Preparation (2nd ed.)

Course Notes and Workbook for Introduction to Sound

Acoustics for the Hearing and Speech Sciences

THIRD EDITION

Charles E. Speaks, Ph.D.
Professor
Monica Ray Zobitz, B.S.
Edward Carney, Ph.D.
Department of Communication Disorders
University of Minnesota
Minneapolis, Minnesota

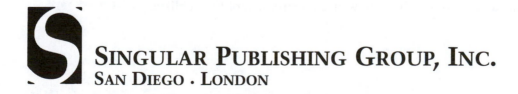
SINGULAR PUBLISHING GROUP, INC.
SAN DIEGO · LONDON

Singular Publishing Group, Inc.
401 West "A" Street, Suite 325
San Diego, California 92101-7904

Singular Publishing Ltd.
19 Compton Terrace
London, N1 2UN, UK

Singular Publishing Group, Inc., publishes textbooks, clinical manuals, clinical reference books, journals, videos, and multimedia materials on speech-language pathology, audiology, otorhinolaryngology, special education, early childhood, aging, occupational therapy, physical therapy, rehabilitation, counseling, mental health, and voice. For your convenience, our entire catalog can be accessed on our website at **http://www.singpub.com**. Our mission to provide you with materials to meet the daily challenges of the ever-changing health care/educational environment will remain on course if we are in touch with you. In that spirit, we welcome your feedback on our products. Please telephone (**1-800-521-8545**), fax (**1-800-774-8398**), or e-mail (**singpub@singpub.com**) your comments and requests to us.

© 1999 by Singular Publishing Group, Inc.

Typeset in 11/13 Trump Mediaeval by So Cal Graphics
Printed in the United States of America by McNaughton and Gunn

All rights, including that of translation, reserved. No part of this publication may be reproduced, stored in a retrieval system, or transmitted in any form or by any means, electronic, mechanical, recording, or otherwise, without the prior written permission of the publisher.

Contents

Preface

Course Notes and Workbook for Introduction to Sound comprises three sections: (1) Course Notes in the form of printed copies of PowerPoint slides; (2) Practice Problems; and (3) Answers to Practice Problems.

Section I: Course Notes. These are printed copies of PowerPoint slides that cover all topics that appear in the third edition of *Introduction to Sound: Acoustics for the Hearing and Speech Sciences*. If Instructors elect to use the slides, which are available on a CD-ROM, during lectures, the printed copy of each slide minimizes the need for students to take copious notes. The printed slides differ from those on the CD-ROM in only one important way. Many of the CD-ROM slides include questions and answers, but *the answers have been omitted in the printed version*. By reading the slides in advance of the lecture, students will have an opportunity to try to formulate the correct answers to those questions independently. Questions without answers are identified by a checkmark located within a square symbol.

Even if the Instructor does not elect to use the CD-ROM for classroom lectures, the printed slides provide a good study guide.

Section II: Practice Problems. Practice Problems contain more than 400 practice problems.

Section III: Answers to Practice Problems. Answers to Practice Problems contains *answers and explanations* of how the correct answers for the practice problems in Section II were obtained.

The *Course Notes and Workbook for Introduction to Sound* are printed on perforated paper that students can tear out and turn in to Instructors. Ideally students should attempt to solve each set of problems as soon as the relevant material has been covered in class. After solving the problems, students can then refer to Answers to Practice Problems to see if their answers are correct, and, if not, how the correct answer should be obtained.

Section I
Course Notes

Course Notes and Workbook for INTRODUCTION TO SOUND: Acoustics for the Hearing and Speech Sciences

Charles Speaks, Monica Ray Zobitz, and Edward Carney

Department of Communication Disorders

University of Minnesota

1999

Technical assistance from Charles Vale

Ch1-1

A Comment About the Printed Slides

All figures and tables in this Course Notes and Workbook also appear in larger, more readable form in the textbook, "Introduction to Sound: Acoustics for the Hearing and Speech Sciences." In the interest of cost and convenience to students, the figures were organized and reproduced in a condensed format in this workbook.

Ch1-2

Chapter 1

THE NATURE OF SOUND WAVES

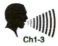

Ch1-3

What is Sound?

- We will emphasize the <u>physical</u>, not <u>psychological</u>, perspective
- A <u>source</u> of sound must be able to <u>vibrate</u>
- To vibrate, a source must have two properties
  - ♦ mass (m)
  - ♦ elasticity (E)

Ch1-4

What is Sound?

- To transmit sound, a medium must be capable of being set into vibration
- To do so, it must have the same two properties
  - ♦ mass (m)
  - ♦ elasticity (E)

Ch1-5

PROPERTIES OF THE TRANSMITTING MEDIUM (EXAMPLE: AIR)

- 400 billion, billion (4×10^{20}) molecules / in.^{3}
- Random molecular motion: 1,500 kph (940 mph)
- Atmospheric pressure:
  - ♦ 14.7 lb / in.^{2}
  - ♦ 100,000 N / m^2
  - ♦ 1,000,000 dynes / cm^2

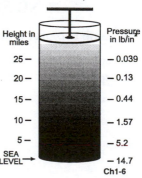

Height in miles	Pressure in lb/in
25 —	— 0.039
20 —	— 0.13
15 —	— 0.44
10 —	— 1.57
5 —	— 5.2
SEA LEVEL→	— 14.7

Ch1-6

Two Physical Properties are Essential

- **What are they?**
  - ☑
  - ☑
- **1. Mass (m)**
  - ♦ **The amount of matter present**
  - ♦ **Applies to gases, liquids, & solids**

Ch1-7

Mass Contrasted with Weight

- **Weight is an attractive gravitational <u>force</u>; mass is the quantity of matter present**
- **160 lb on earth = 27 lb on the moon because force of gravity is 6:1**
- **Weight ∝ to mass, but they are different concepts**
  - ♦ **weight is a force**
  - ♦ **mass is the quantity of matter present**
  - ♦ **air has mass and weight**

Ch1-8

Mass (m) and Density (ρ)

- **Density (ρ) is the mass per unit volume ($\rho = m/v$)**
- **Density is a quantity <u>derived</u> from another quantity (mass)**
- **Note how density varies with height above sea level**

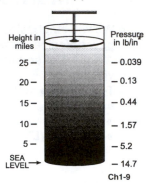

Height in miles	Pressure in lb/in
25 —	— 0.039
20 —	— 0.13
15 —	— 0.44
10 —	— 1.57
5 —	— 5.2
SEA LEVEL→	— 14.7

Ch1-9

Two Physical Properties

- **2. Elasticity (E)**
  - ♦ **Property that enables <u>recovery</u> from <u>distortion</u> of shape or volume**
  - ♦ **Concept of "Elastic Limit"**
  - ♦ **Air: "Tendency of air volume to return to its former volume after compression" i.e., density is restored**

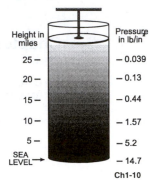

Height in miles	Pressure in lb/in
25 —	— 0.039
20 —	— 0.13
15 —	— 0.44
10 —	— 1.57
5 —	— 5.2
SEA LEVEL→	— 14.7

Ch1-10

PROPERTIES OF THE SOUND SOURCE

- **Same two properties: What are they?**
  - ☑
  - ☑

Ch1-11

Vibratory Motion of a Tuning Fork

- **Animation F1-2**
- **Strike the fork: Vibration occurs**
- **Tines displaced from equilibrium**
- **Amplitude of displacement is proportional to force applied**

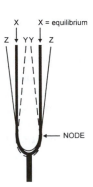

Ch1-12

Newton's First Law of Motion: Inertia

- The property addressed by Newton's first law is called <u>inertia</u>
- Newton's Inertial Law: All bodies remain at rest or in a state of uniform motion unless another force acts in opposition
- Magnitude of inertia is directly proportional to the <u>mass</u>: thus mass is a <u>measure of inertia</u>

Ch1-13

Vibratory Motion: Why does it occur?

- The interaction of two opposing forces: inertia and elasticity
- Back and forth, to and fro, movement
- The opposition of two forces is consistent with Newton's third law

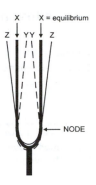

Ch1-14

Newton's Third Law of Motion: Reaction Forces

- Newton's Third Law: With every force there <u>must</u> be an <u>equal</u> and opposite reaction force
  - ♦ Hammer- nail: Bat- ball
  - ♦ Force cannot exist alone
- Vibration: elasticity is the <u>reaction force</u> to inertia
  - ♦ Vibration continues without reapplication of external force: vibration sustained by opposing forces
  - ♦ One <u>cycle of vibration</u> (return to #14)

Ch1-15

SOUND SOURCE ACTING ON A MEDIUM

- Animation F1-3
- Place tuning fork in medium: observe effect on medium
- Before force is applied, particles are, on average, equidistant from one another

Ch1-16

Movement of Air Particles

- Particles move about positions of equilibrium because of two opposing forces: What are they?
  ☑
  ☑

Ch1-17

Movement of Air Particles

- Force from A to B to..........n
  - ♦ Across rows: particles move to and fro <u>over a small distance</u>
  - ♦ Note <u>crowding</u> (compression) and <u>thinning</u> (rarefaction)

Ch1-18

Movement of Air Mass

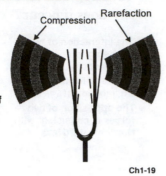

- Animation F1-4
- Density increases: <u>compression</u>
- Density decreases: <u>rarefaction</u>
- Alternate regions of compression and rarefaction move through medium

Ch1-19

Displacement of Air Medium & Wave Motion

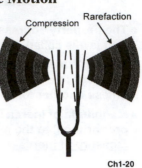

- Medium is <u>not displaced</u> over a great distance!
- A wave of disturbance moves through the medium
  - ♦ Sporting events (the "wave")
  - ♦ Synchronized flashing of light bulbs on theater marquees

Ch1-20

Displacement of Air Medium & Wave Motion

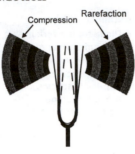

- SOUND: <u>characterized</u> by propagation of density changes through elastic medium
- Need to consider selected physical quantities such as
  - ♦ mass
  - ♦ density
  - ♦ force
  - ♦ pressure
  - ♦ displacement

Ch1-21

FUNDAMENTAL PHYSICAL QUANTITIES

- There are three: What are they?

  ☑

  ☑

  ☑

- All other physical quantities are derived

Ch1-22

Systems of Measure

- Metric: <u>MKS</u> & cgs
- English: fps

	MKS	cgs	fps
♦ length	(m)	(cm)	(ft)
♦ mass	(kg)	(g)	(lb)
♦ time	(s)	(s)	(s)

Ch1-23

1. Length

- A measure of distance: the amount of spatial separation between two points
  - ♦ How many times a unit (meter, cm, ft, etc.) is contained in a given distance.
  - ♦ 1 m = distance traveled by light in a vacuum during 3×10^{-9} ms.

Ch1-24

Units of Measure: Length

- Units of Measure

  MKS -- meter (m)

  cgs -- centimeter (cm)

  fps -- foot (ft)

- Sample Conversions

  1 in. = 2.54 cm

  1 ft = .3048 m

  1 m = 100 cm

  1 cm = .01 m

  1 mm = .001 m

  Ch1-25

2. Mass

- The quantity of matter present
- Defines the magnitude of <u>inertia</u>
- Inertia ∝ mass
  - A steel ball and ping-pong ball are the same size: Which has greater mass, hence greater inertia?
    ☑

  Ch1-26

Units of Measure: Mass

- MKS ----- kilogram (kg)
- cgs ----- gram (g)
- fps ----- pound (lb)
- The quantity of mass defines the <u>amount of inertia</u>

  Ch1-27

3. Time

- A quantity expressed in seconds (s), minutes (min), hours (hr), etc.
- 1 s = 1/86,400 of a solar day
  - 24 hrs × 60 min × 60 s = 86,400

  Ch1-28

Units of Measure: Time

- MKS ---- second (s)
- cgs ---- second (s)
- fps ---- second (s)

  Ch1-29

DERIVED PHYSICAL QUANTITIES

- A derived quantity is a <u>quotient</u> or <u>product</u> of fundamental, or of fundamental and derived, physical quantities
- Example: length vs. area

  3 m

  2 m

  - L_l = 3 m fundamental quantity
  - L_w = 2 m fundamental quantity
  - A = 6 m^2 derived quantity

  Ch1-30

Derived Quantities of Interest

- Displacement **(x)**
- Velocity   **(c)**
- Acceleration   **(a)**
- Force   **(F)**
- Pressure   **(p)**

Ch1-31

1. Displacement (x)

- A change in position (re: equilibrium, e.g.)

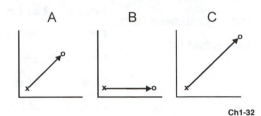

Ch1-32

1. Displacement (x)

- A <u>vector</u> quantity: incorporates both
  - ♦ <u>Magnitude</u>
  - ♦ <u>Direction</u>
    - \>> A vs. B
    - \>> A vs. C
    - \>> B vs. C
- Contrast with a <u>scalar</u> quantity: has only <u>magnitude</u> (e.g., mass, time, energy, etc.)

A   B   C

Ch1-33

2. Velocity (c)

- The <u>amount of displacement per unit time</u>

  Or
- The <u>time-rate of displacement</u>
- Also a vector quantity
- Average velocity
  - ♦ c = x / t
  - ♦ c = derived (x) / fundamental (t)

Ch1-34

Velocity (c) vs. Speed (s)

- Speed is a scalar quantity (only <u>magnitude</u>)
- s = d / t
- $c_{resultant} = \sqrt{s_1{}^2 + s_2{}^2}$
- Average vs. Instantaneous Velocity

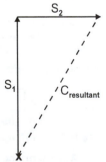

Ch1-35

Summary of Velocity: Displacement Per Unit Time

- MKS --- m / s

- cgs --- cm / s

- fps --- ft / s, mph, etc.

Ch1-36

3. Acceleration (a)

- The <u>time-rate change in velocity</u>
- Also a <u>vector quantity</u>
- Positive vs. Negative Acceleration (Deceleration)

3. Acceleration (a)

- $a = \Delta c/t = (c_2 - c_1)/t$
  - $c_1 = 20$ m/s
  - $c_2 = 40$ m/s
  - $t = 5$ s
  - What is a?
  - ☑

3. Acceleration (a)

- A car moves around a circular tract at a constant <u>speed</u>. Is it accelerating?
  - ☑

4. Force (F)

- A push or pull
- The product of mass (m) and acceleration (a)
- F = ma (Newton's 2nd Law: a = F/m)
- Object has mass (inertia), which opposes change in motion: force is applied to overcome inertia
  - $a = F/m$
  - $\therefore F = ma$

Consequences of Force

- Distortion of matter
  and / or
- Acceleration of matter
- A push or pull <u>OR</u> that which imparts acceleration to a mass

Force as a Vector

- Magnitude and Direction
- Vector addition necessary
  - If two forces are at right angles to one another, resultant forces solved by the Pythagorean theorem
  - $F_{resultant} = \sqrt{F_1^2 + F_2^2}$

Units of Measure of Force

- MKS — newton (N)
  - ◆ Force required to accelerate a mass of 1 kg from c = 0 m/s to c = 1 m/s in 1 s
- cgs — dyne
  - ◆ Force required to accelerate mass of 1g from c = 0 cm/s to c = 1 cm/s in 1 s
- 1 N = 100,000 dynes

Ch1-43

5. Pressure (p)

- Force per unit area
- $p = F / A$
- $p = 1\,N / 100\,m^2$
  $= .01\,N / m^2$

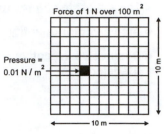

Ch1-44

Units of Measure of Pressure

- What are they in MKS and cgs systems?
  - ☑
  - ☑
- $1\,N / m^2$ = how many dynes / cm^2?
  - ♦ $1\,N / m^2 = 10$ dynes / cm^2

Ch1-45

Derivation

$1\,N = 100,000$ dynes
$1\,m = 100\,cm$
Thus,
$1\,N/m^2 = 100,000$ dynes/m^2
$\quad m^2 = m \times m$
$1\,N/m^2 = 100,000$ dynes/$10,000\,cm^2$
Thus,
$\quad 1\,N/m^2 = 10$ dynes/cm^2

Ch1-46

An Alternative Unit of Measure for Pressure

- The pascal (Pa)
- 1 pascal (Pa) = $1\,N/m^2$
- 1 Pa = how many dynes / cm^2?
  - ☑

Ch1-47

VIBRATORY MOTION OF A SPRING - MASS SYSTEM

- Animation F1-8
- Panel A: spring at equilibrium
- Panel B: spring compressed
- Panel C: spring stretched

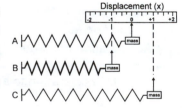

Ch1-48

Characteristics of a Spring

- Spring can be <u>compressed</u>
- Elasticity (<u>restoring force</u>) opposes deformation force

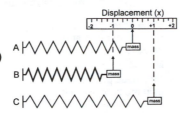

Ch1-49

Characteristics of a Spring

- Hooke's Law: Magnitude of restoring force (F_r) is directly proportional to magnitude of displacement (x)
- $F_r = -kx$
- As spring is compressed, greater force required for additional compression

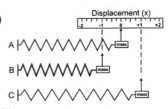

Ch1-50

Stiffness and Compliance

- Stiffness is the spring constant (k)
- Compliance is the inverse of stiffness

Ch1-51

VIBRATORY MOTION OF A SPRING - MASS SYSTEM

- Displace mass
- Spring is compressed
- System is set into vibration

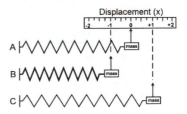

Ch1-52

VIBRATORY MOTION OF A SPRING - MASS SYSTEM

- Vibration sustained by interaction of two opposing forces: What are they?
- ☑
- ☑
- System engages in <u>simple harmonic</u>, or <u>sinusoidal</u>, <u>motion</u>

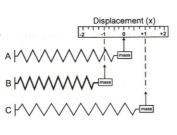

Ch1-53

THE PENDULUM: EXAMPLE OF SLOW MOTION VIBRATION

- Animation F1-9
- Restoring force <u>opposes</u> applied force
- Restoring force is gravity, not elasticity
- Sustained vibratory motion has two opposing forces:
  - ◆ Inertia
  - ◆ Gravity

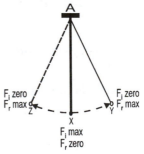

Ch1-54

THE PENDULUM: EXAMPLE OF SLOW MOTION VIBRATION

- Inertial force (F_i) is maximal at equilibrium and zero at maximum displacement where motion is momentarily halted
- Restoring force (F_r) is maximal at maximum displacement and zero at equilibrium

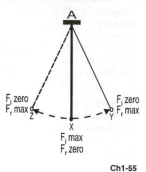

Ch1-55

Momentum
Effect of momentum replaces force of inertia

- Momentum given by the product of mass and velocity
- $M = mc$
- Why does pendulum gain momentum as it approaches equilibrium?
- ☑

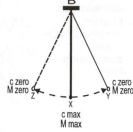

Ch1-56

Momentum
Effect of momentum replaces force of inertia

- c is maximal at equilibrium and zero at maximum displacement where motion is momentarily halted
- M is also maximal at equilibrium and zero at maximum displacement where motion is momentarily halted

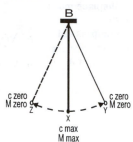

Ch1-57

The Energy Principle

- Used to describe vibratory motion of a pendulum
- System must receive a supply of energy
- Energy is something that can <u>produce a change in matter</u>
  - ♦ e.g., Displacement, distortion

Ch1-58

The Energy Principle

- If a change in matter occurs, <u>work</u> has been done
- Energy is the <u>capacity to do work</u>

Ch1-59

Energy vs. Work

- Energy: Something that a body <u>possesses</u>
- Work: Something that a body <u>does</u>

Ch1-60

Work

- A body is moved because a force is applied

- Work is given by product of the force applied and the distance moved

$$W = Fd$$

Units of Measure: Work

- MKS — joule
- How would you define it?
  - ☑
- cgs — erg
- How would you define it?
  - ☑

Units of Measure: Work

- 1 joule = 10^7 ergs
- Derivation
  - ♦ 10^0 N = 10^5 dynes
  - ♦ 10^0 m = 10^2 cm
  - ♦ 10^5 dynes $\times 10^2$ cm = 10^7 ergs

Transformation of Energy

The unifying concept that explains SHM and pendular motion, even though RESTORING FORCES are different

- Energy is not depleted; It is transferred or transformed
- Potential Energy (PE)
  - ♦ Stored energy
- Kinetic Energy (KE)
  - ♦ Energy of motion
- PE + KE = k

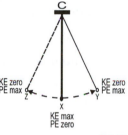

Transformation of Energy

- KE is
  - ♦ maximal at equilibrium where c is maximal, &
  - ♦ zero at maximum displacement where motion is momentarily halted and c = 0
- PE is
  - ♦ maximal at maximum displacement, &
  - ♦ zero at equilibrium

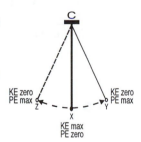

Frictional Resistance

- Motion ultimately ceases because of frictional resistance

- Frictional resistance is a <u>force</u> that opposes motion and thus limits velocity

Frictional Resistance

- **KE transformed to <u>thermal energy</u> (heat)**
- **Result is damping, or damped vibration**
- **Frictional resistance is analogous to electrical resistance to the flow of current in a circuit**

Ch1-67

Characteristics of Pendular Motion

- **1. Amplitude of displacement**
  - ◆ **A vector quantity**
  - ◆ **Why a vector?**
  - ☑

Ch1-68

Characteristics of Pendular Motion

- **2. Frequency (f)**
  - ◆ **The rate of vibratory motion**
  - ◆ **The number of "cycles per second" (cps)**
  - ◆ **Unit of measure: hertz (Hz)**
  - ◆ **1 Hz = 1 cps**

Ch1-69

Characteristics of Pendular Motion

- **What defines "one cycle?"**
  - ☑

Ch1-70

Characteristics of Pendular Motion

- **3. Period (T)**
  - ◆ **The time required to complete one cycle**
  - ◆ **(seconds per cycle)**
  - ◆ **Equations !**
    - ≫ **T = 1 / f**
    - ≫ **f = 1 / T** ⟩ **Reciprocal relations**

Ch1-71

Determinants of Frequency: Pendulum

- $T = 2\pi\sqrt{L/G}$
  - ◆ $T \propto \sqrt{L}$
  - ◆ $T \propto 1/\sqrt{G}$
  - ◆ **G = 9.8 m / s² (on earth)**

Ch1-72

Determinants of Frequency: Pendulum

- f = ?
  - ☑

- What are the proportional relations of f with L and G?
  - ☑

  - ☑

PROPORTIONALITY

- **Inversely proportional**
  - ◆ A ∝ 1 / B
- **Directly Proportional**
  - ◆ A ∝ B

Examples

- $T = 2\pi\sqrt{L/G}$: What are the proportional relations of T with L and G?
  - ☑
  - ☑
- W = Fd: What are the proportional relations of W with F and d?
  - ☑
  - ☑

SOUND WAVE PROPAGATION

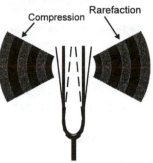

- Air particles move over a very small distance
  - ◆ 7.68×10^{-8} m
  - ◆ Equal to 1 / 300 of the diameter of a hydrogen molecule

SOUND WAVE PROPAGATION

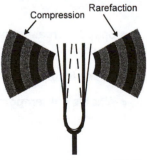

- See alternate regions of compression (increased density) and rarefaction (decreased density)
- That <u>disturbance</u> is propagated through the medium

SOUND WAVE PROPAGATION

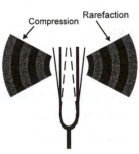

- Consider water analogy
  - ◆ Place cork on water surface and initiate a wave
  - ◆ wave (crests and troughs) move by the cork
  - ◆ cork bobs (approximately) upward and downward

Two Events That Occur at Some Rate

- Rate (frequency) of vibratory movement

- Rate (speed) of wave propagation

Frequency of Vibratory Motion (f)

- Frequency of vibration of the source is determined by characteristics of <u>source</u>!
  - ◆ Tuning fork: density of metal & length of bar
  - ◆ String or wire: length, cross-sectional mass, & tension
- Frequency of vibration of <u>air particles</u> is the same as frequency of the source!

Speed of Sound (s)

- Speed of wave propagation is governed by properties of the <u>medium</u>!
- Examples
  - ◆ Light   299,728,458   m / s
    186,282.397   mi / s
  - ◆ Sound   331   m / s
    1085.96   ft / s
  - \>> At sea level, and
  - \>> If temperature = 0° C

Speed of Sound in Air

- $s = \sqrt{E/\rho}$
- What are the proportional relations of s with E and ρ?
  - ☑
  - ☑

Speed of Sound in Air

- Elasticity: Units of measure
  - ◆ MKS: N/m^2
  - ◆ cgs: $dynes/cm^2$
- Density (mass / volume): Units of measure
  - ◆ MKS: kg/m^3
  - ◆ cgs: g/cm^3

Effects of "Temperature"

- Speed increases by 0.61 m/s (2 ft/s) for each 1° C increase in temperature
- At sea level, at 0° C, s = 331 m/s
- What is <u>s</u> if temperature = 20° C?
  - ☑

Speed of Sound for Different Transmitting Media

- Air: 331 m/s or 1,086 ft/s
- Water: about 4 times that of air
          (1,433 m/s)
- Steel: about 14 times that of air
          (4,704 m/s)

Ch1-85

Steel Compared to Air

- Steel is 6,000 times more dense than air
  - $s \propto 1/\sqrt{\rho}$, but
- Steel is 1,230,000 times more elastic than air
  - $s \propto \sqrt{E}$

Ch1-86

Steel Compared to Air

- $\sqrt{1{,}230{,}000 / 6{,}000} = 14.3$
  - $\sqrt{(1.23 \times 10^6) / (6 \times 10^3)} = 1.43 \times 10^1$
- Elasticity: Best defined as the ability to <u>resist</u> deformation!

Ch1-87

TYPES OF WAVE MOTION

- Classified by direction of <u>vibration of medium</u> re: direction of <u>wave propagation</u>
- Two types of wave motion
  - Transverse
  - Longitudinal

Ch1-88

Transverse Wave Motion

- Stretched rope or string
- Animation F1- 10
- Vibration of medium is 90° re: direction of wave propagation
  - Elements of rope move up & down
  - Wave moves at right angles
  - Note peaks and valleys

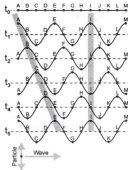

Ch1-89

Longitudinal Wave Motion

- Spring-mass system
- Animation F1-11
- Direction of particle movement is parallel to wave movement
  - Elements of spring move back & forth
  - Wave moves in same plane
  - Note compressions and rarefactions

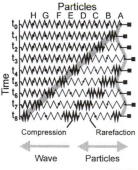

Ch1-90

SOUND WAVES

- They are longitudinal waves
- Particles oscillate about their equilibrium positions
- Wave is propagated in same plane as particle displacement

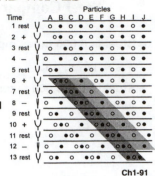

Ch1-91

TRANSFER OF ENERGY

- Sound is <u>characterized</u> as propagation of density changes through an elastic medium
- Sound is <u>defined</u> as transfer of energy through an elastic medium
  - ♦ Energy is transferred in direction wave is propagated
  - ♦ Air mass offers <u>resistance</u>
  - ♦ Kinetic energy is transformed to thermal energy

Ch1-92

Chapter 2

SIMPLE HARMONIC MOTION

Review: Spring-Mass System

- Hooke's Law
  - ◆ Magnitude of restoring force is proportional to distance displaced
  - ◆ $F_r \propto x$
- Does the magnitude of restoring force change over time?
  ☑

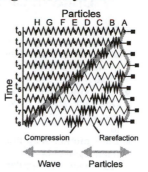

Review: Spring-Mass System

- Result: vibration or oscillation of system
- Magnitude of displacement (x) changes over time: 0, +, 0, -, 0, etc.
- One cycle
- Note the shape of displacement path of the mass
- System engages in simple harmonic motion

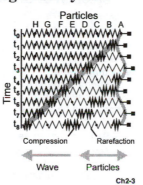

THE WAVEFORM

- Waveform shows change in <u>some quantity</u> as a function of time; e.g.,
  - ◆ Displacement   (x)
  - ◆ Velocity   (c)
  - ◆ Acceleration   (a)
  - ◆ Force   (F)
  - ◆ Pressure   (p)
  - ◆ Momentum, etc.   (M)

THE WAVEFORM

- A plot of change in amplitude of displacement (x) over time
- The display is called the <u>time-domain waveform</u>, or <u>waveform</u>
- Air does not actually undergo this form of excursion: the waveform is a <u>representation</u>

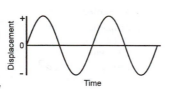

THE CONCEPT OF SIMPLE HARMONIC MOTION

- Spring-mass system undergoes simple harmonic motion
- SHM is characterized as projected uniform circular motion

Uniform Circular Motion

- A point (dot) moves about the circumference of a circle at a constant number of degrees of rotation per second
- "Dot" engages in SHM
- One cycle equals how many degrees? ☑
- But -- motion of spring-mass system is <u>rectilinear</u>, not circular

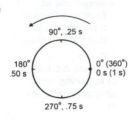

Ch2-7

Degrees vs. Linear Displacement

- Animation F2-3
- Wall is stationary
  - ◆ Circular motion projected as rectilinear (straight-line) motion

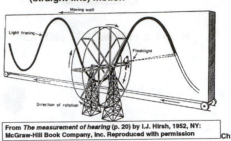

From *The measurement of hearing* (p. 20) by I.J. Hirsh, 1952, NY: McGraw-Hill Book Company, Inc. Reproduced with permission   Ch2-8

Degrees vs. Linear Displacement

- Wall moves from right to left
  - ◆ The waveform of SHM is projected

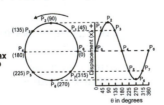

From *The measurement of hearing* (p. 20) by I.J. Hirsh, 1952, NY: McGraw-Hill Book Company, Inc. Reproduced with permission   -9

Projection of Uniform Circular Motion

- Animation F2-4
- Display is called a <u>displacement waveform</u>
- Compare what happens between 45° and 90° with what happened between 0° and 45°
  - ◆ Same # of degrees
  - ◆ Magnitude of linear displacement above baseline is different

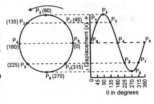

Ch2-10

Projection of Uniform Circular Motion

- Displacement and degrees of rotation
  - ◆ 90° and 270° correspond to x_{max}
  - ◆ 0°, 180°, and 360° correspond to equilibrium
  - ◆ Rotation through 360° equals one cycle

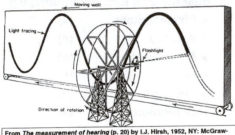

Ch2-11

The Sine Wave

- Animation 2-5
- Projections from three wheels of different sizes
  - ◆ Each projection has the same shape
  - ◆ The unifying constant is the sine of the angle

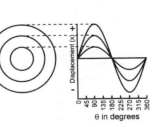

Ch2-12

Sine of an Angle

- **The ratio x/r is a <u>constant</u> for any given angle**
  - ◆ **x/r: the <u>sine of the angle</u>**
  - ◆ **b/r: the <u>cosine of the angle</u>**
  - ◆ **x/b: the <u>tangent of the angle</u>**

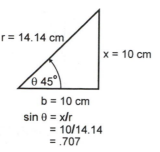

$$\sin\theta = x/r$$
$$= 10/14.14$$
$$= .707$$

Ch2-13

Sine of an Angle

- **When x = 10 and r = 14.14, x/r = .707: sin 45° = .707**
- **Suppose x = 20 and r = 28.28, but θ = 45°: What is sin θ?**
  - ☑
- **For a given angle, e.g., 45°, sin θ is a constant regardless of the lengths of x and r**

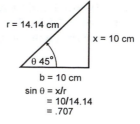

$$\sin\theta = x/r$$
$$= 10/14.14$$
$$= .707$$

Ch2-14

Sine of an Angle

- **Suppose r remains 14.14, but x = 5.41 and θ = 22.5°: What is sine θ?**
  - ☑
- **Thus, sin θ is different for different angles**

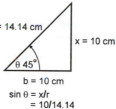

$$\sin\theta = x/r$$
$$= 10/14.14$$
$$= .707$$

Ch2-15

Sines of Sample Angles

Angle	Sine
0	0
45	0.707
90	1
135	0.707
180	0
225	-0.707
270	-1
315	-0.707
360	0

	θ	sinθ
A	45	.707
B	45	.707
C	45	.707

Ch2-16

Displacement (x) Replaced By Sine of the Angle

- **Height of each projection now is the <u>sine of the angle</u> (sin θ), not x**
- **Three projections now superimposed on one another. Why?**
  - ☑

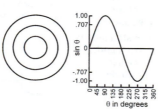

Ch2-17

Construction of a Sine Wave

Table 2-1. Sines of selected angles at 11.25° intervals

θ	sin θ	θ	sin θ	θ	sin θ	θ	sin θ
0.00	0.000						
11.25	.195	101.25	.981	191.25	-.195	281.25	-.981
22.50	.383	112.50	.924	202.50	-.383	292.50	-.924
33.75	.556	123.75	.831	213.75	-.556	303.75	-.831
45.00	.707	135.00	.707	225.00	-.707	315.00	-.707
56.25	.831	146.25	.556	236.25	-.831	326.25	-.556
67.50	.924	157.50	.383	247.50	-.924	337.50	-.383
78.75	.981	168.75	.195	258.75	-.981	348.75	-.195
90.00	1.000	180.00	.000	270.00	-1.000	360.00	0.000

- **Sin θ for angles at equal intervals of 11.25° from 0° to 360°**

Ch2-18

Construction of a Sine Wave

● In the next slide each value of sin θ
in Table 2-1 is plotted as a function
of θ: What will the function look like?
☑

Ch2-19

Construction of a Sine Wave

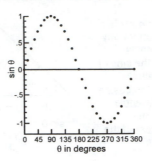

Ch2-20

Summary of Sinusoidal Motion

● Common element: sine of the angle
● The sine of the angle corresponds to
<u>percentage of maximum displacement</u>:
  ♦ At 22.5°,   sin θ = .383: 38.3% of x_{max}
  ♦ At 45°,   sin θ = .707: 70.7% of x_{max}
  ♦ At 90°,   sin θ = 1.00: 100% of x_{max}
  ♦ and so forth

Ch2-21

Summary of Sinusoidal Motion

● Thus, SHM can be called sinusoidal
motion
● Projection of sinusoidal motion is
called a sine wave, or sinusoidal
wave

Ch2-22

Rectilinear Motion Shown as Uniform Circular Motion

● How can back &
forth motion be
represented as
uniform circular
motion?
● Animation F2- 9

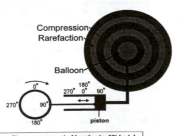

Adapted from *The measurement of hearing* (p. 22) by I.J.
Hirsh, 1952, NY: McGraw-Hill Book Company, Inc.
Reproduced with permission.

Ch2-23

Rectilinear Motion Shown as Uniform Circular Motion

● Wheel rotates
clockwise
(circular motion)
  ♦ Piston moves
  back and
  forth in
  cylinder
  (rectilinear
  motion)

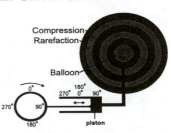

Adapted from *The measurement of hearing* (p. 22) by I.J.
Hirsh, 1952, NY: McGraw-Hill Book Company, Inc.
Reproduced with permission.

Ch2-24

Rectilinear Motion Shown as Uniform Circular Motion

♦ Points along rectilinear excursion of piston labeled in degrees to correspond to points along circular excursion of wheel

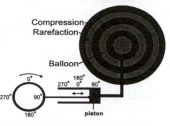

Adapted from *The measurement of hearing* (p. 22) by I.J. Hirsh, 1952, NY: McGraw-Hill Book Company, Inc. Reproduced with permission.

Ch2-25

Simple Harmonic Motion and Sound Waves

● At 0°, balloon is partially inflated
● At 90°, balloon maximally inflated
● At 270°, balloon minimally inflated
● Compressions and rarefactions are propagated through medium
● The result is a sound wave

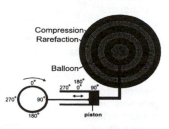

Adapted from *The measurement of hearing* (p. 22) by I.J. Hirsh, 1952, NY: McGraw-Hill Book Company, Inc. Reproduced with permission.

Ch2-26

DIMENSIONS OF THE SINE WAVE

● Five dimensions of sine waves
♦ Amplitude
♦ Frequency
♦ Period
♦ Phase
♦ Wavelength

Ch2-27

DIMENSIONS OF THE SINE WAVE

● (1) AMPLITUDE
● Note phasic relations among:
♦ displacement
♦ velocity
♦ acceleration
♦ pressure

Adapted from *The measurement of hearing* (p. 24) by I.J. Hirsh, 1952, NY: McGraw-Hill Book Company, Inc. Reproduced with permission.

Ch2-28

Amplitude

● Particle velocity leads particle displacement by 90°: Why?
☑

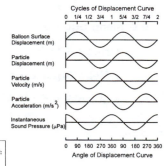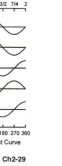

Adapted from *The measurement of hearing* (p. 24) by I.J. Hirsh, 1952, NY: McGraw-Hill Book Company, Inc. Reproduced with permission.

Ch2-29

Amplitude

● Particle acceleration leads particle displacement by 180°: Why?
♦ $F_i = ma$ (Newton's 2nd Law)
♦ $F_r = -kx$ (Hooke's Law)
♦ $F_i = F_r$ (Newton's 3rd Law)
♦ $ma = -kx$

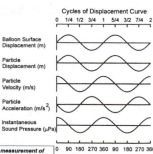

Adapted from *The measurement of hearing* (p. 24) by I.J. Hirsh, 1952, NY: McGraw-Hill Book Company, Inc. Reproduced with permission.

Ch2-30

Amplitude

- ♦ m and -k are constants
- ♦ a and x are variables
- ♦ a and x must be opposites (Newton's 3rd Law)
- ● Instantaneous sound pressure "mirrors" particle velocity and leads particle displacement by 90°

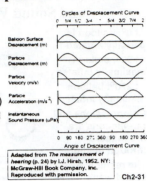

Adapted from *The measurement of hearing* (p. 24) by I.J. Hirsh, 1952. NY: McGraw-Hill Book Company, Inc. Reproduced with permission.   Ch2-31

Amplitude

- ● a. Instantaneous Amplitude (a)
- ● b. Maximum Amplitude (A)
- ● c. Peak-to-Peak Amplitude
- ● d. Root-Mean-Square Amplitude (rms)

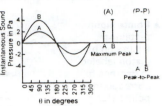

Ch2-32

Concept of rms

- ● Sampling the waveform: $X_1 ... X_6$
- ● Compute standard deviation, σ
- ● rms is standard deviation of all instantaneous amplitudes
- ● rms: the square <u>root</u> (r) of the <u>mean</u> (m) of the <u>squared</u> (s) deviations of instantaneous values

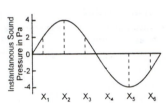

Ch2-33

Concept of rms

- ● rms ↔ σ
- ● rms² ↔ σ²

Table 2-2. Procedures for calculating the standard deviation

X	$X - \overline{X}$	$(X - \overline{X})^2$
2.0	2.0	4.0
4.0	4.0	16.0
2.0	2.0	4.0
-2.0	-2.0	4.0
-4.0	-4.0	16.0
-2.0	-2.0	4.0
$\sum X = 0.0$		$\sum (X - \overline{X})^2 = 48.0$

$$\frac{\sum X}{N} = 0.0 \quad \sigma^2 = \frac{\sum (X - \overline{X})^2}{N} = 8.0 \text{ (ms)}$$

$$\sigma = \sqrt{\frac{\sum (X - \overline{X})^2}{N}} = 2.828 \text{ (rms)}$$

Calculation of rms for a Sine Wave

- ● rms = $A / \sqrt{2}$
- ● rms = A / 1.414
  = A (1 / 1.414)
- ● rms = A (.707)

Ch2-35

Amplitude

- ● e. Mean Square
  - ♦ rms = $A / \sqrt{2}$
  - ♦ Mean Square = rms²
  - ♦ Mean Square = $A^2 / 2$

Ch2-36

Amplitude

- **f. Full-Wave Rectified Average (FW$_{AVG}$)**
  - ♦ Arithmetic mean of all instantaneous amplitudes in the rectified wave
  - ♦ FW$_{AVG}$ = 2A / π
    = 2A / 3.1416
    = A (.636)

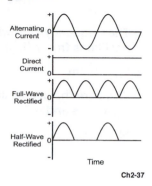

Ch2-37

Amplitude

- **g. Half-Wave Rectified Average (HW$_{AVG}$)**
  - ♦ HW$_{AVG}$ = A / π
    = A / 3.1416
    = A (.318)

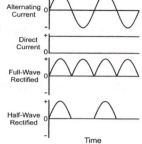

Ch2-38

Comparison Among Metrics

- **Instantaneous values vary sinusoidally over time**
- **Other values are time-averaged**

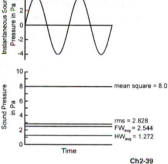

mean square = 8.0

rms = 2.828
FW$_{avg}$ = 2.544
HW$_{avg}$ = 1.272

Ch2-39

DIMENSIONS OF THE SINE WAVE

- **(2) FREQUENCY (f)**
  - ♦ **The rate, in Hz, at which a sinusoid repeats itself**
- **(3) PERIOD (T)**
  - ♦ **The time required to complete one cycle**
- **f = 1/T; T = 1/f**

Ch2-40

Relation Between Frequency and Period

- **T of X = .001 s: f = ?**
  - ☑
- **T of Y = .0005 s: f = ?**
  - ☑

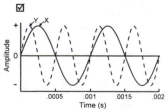

Ch2-41

Units of Measure For Frequency and Period

- **Frequency (f)**
  - ♦ **Hz to kHz: Divide by 1,000**
  - ♦ **kHz to Hz: Multiply by 1,000**
- **Period (T)**
  - ♦ **s to ms: Multiply by 1,000**
  - ♦ **ms to s: Divide by 1,000**
- **f = 1/T and T = 1/f**

Table 2-3. Standard units of measure for frequency and period

FREQUENCY		MULTIPLIER	PERIOD		MULTIPLIER
Hertz	(Hz)	1	second	(s)	1
Kilohertz	(kHz)	1,000	millisecond	(ms)	.001
Megahertz	(MHz)	1,000,000	microsecond	(μs)	.000001
Gigahertz	(GHz)	1,000,000,000	nanosecond	(ns)	.000000001

Ch2-42

Determinants of Frequency

- Frequency depends on <u>properties of the source</u> of sound

- Spring-mass system: <u>mass</u> (m) and <u>stiffness</u> (s) of system

Ch2-43

Natural Frequency (f_{nat})

- The frequency with which a system oscillates freely (f_{nat})

- $f_{nat} = \sqrt{s/m}$

- What are the proportional relations of f_{nat} with s and m?

  ☑

  ☑

Ch2-44

f_{nat} of Vibrating String

- $f = 1/2L\sqrt{t/m}$

- What are the proportional relations of f_{nat} with L, t, and m?

  ☑

  ☑

  ☑

Ch2-45

Angular Velocity (ω)

- Alternative ways to express frequency
  - degrees / s; circle divided into 360 equal parts
    - >> 1 Hz = 360°/s; 10 Hz = 3600°/s
  - quarter cycles / s; circle divided into 4 equal parts
    - >> 1 Hz = 4 quarter cycles / s;
      10 Hz = 40 quarter cycles / s

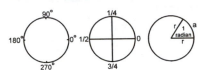

Ch2-46

Angular Velocity (ω)

- The measure of choice
  - 2π radians / s; circle divided into 2π (6.2832) equal parts
    - >> 1 Hz = 2π radians / s
- An angle = 1 radian when intersection of 2 sides of angle with C yields arc with length = to radius

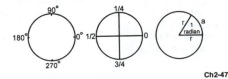

Ch2-47

Comments on the Radian

- 1 radian = 57.3°
  - 360° / 57.3° = 2π
  - Thus, 360° = $2\pi r$
- Snip a circle: unroll it
  - For circles of all sizes:
  - Length = 2π (6.2832) times radius of circle ($2\pi r$)

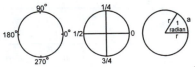

Ch2-48

Comments on the Radian

- One cycle = 360°
    - 360° = 2π radians
    - 360°/s = 2π radians/s
- $\omega = 2\pi f$

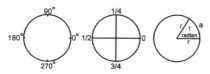

Ch2-49

DIMENSIONS OF THE SINE WAVE

- (4) PHASE
    - Four reference points: A, B, C, & D

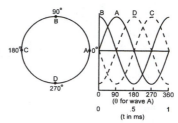

Ch2-50

Phase

- At moment rotation begins, what is displacement in degrees for each of four points?
    - ☑ A =
    - ☑ B =
    - ☑ C =
    - ☑ D =

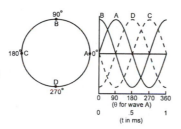

Ch2-51

Starting Phase

- That defines the starting phase; the angle, in degrees, at the moment rotation begins

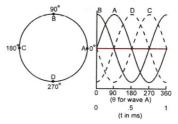

Ch2-52

Starting Phase

- Starting phase relations
    - B leads A by?
        - ☑
    - C leads B by?
        - ☑
    - C leads A by?
        - ☑
    - D leads B by?
        - ☑
    - B lags C by?
        - ☑

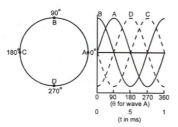

Ch2-53

Instantaneous Phase

- Angle of rotation at some specified moment in time
- What are phase angles at t = .5 ms?
    - ☑ A =
    - ☑ B =
    - ☑ C =
    - ☑ D =

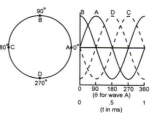

Ch2-54

Phase Angles in Radians

- Radians replace degrees on abscissa
- $360^\circ = 2\pi$ radians
- $0^\circ = ?$
  - ☑
- $90^\circ = ?$
  - ☑
- $180^\circ = ?$
  - ☑
- $270^\circ = ?$
  - ☑

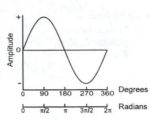

Ch2-55

DIMENSIONS OF THE SINE WAVE

- (5) WAVELENGTH (λ)
- Two quantities are measured with respect to <u>time</u>
  - ◆ Frequency (f)
  - ◆ Speed of sound (s)

Ch2-56

Wavelength

- Wavelength (λ) relates frequency and speed of sound
- λ = distance traveled during one period
- $\lambda = s / f$
- What are the proportional relations of λ with s and f?
  - ☑
  - ☑

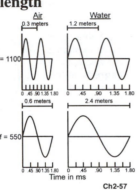

Ch2-57

Wavelength

- Examples
  - ◆ In air: f = 1100 Hz, s = 340 m / s; $\lambda = ?$
    - ☑
  - ◆ In air: f = 550 Hz, s = 340 m / s; $\lambda = ?$
    - ☑

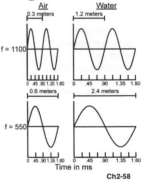

Ch2-58

Wavelength

- ◆ In water: f = 1100 Hz, s = 1360 m / s; $\lambda = ?$
  - ☑
- ◆ In water: f = 550 Hz, s = 1360 m / s; $\lambda = ?$
  - ☑

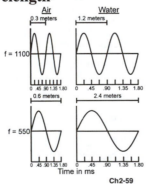

Ch2-59

DAMPING

- Oscillating systems encounter opposition to motion: <u>friction</u>, or <u>frictional resistance</u>
- Friction limits velocity

Ch2-60

Review of SHM and Important Phasic Relations

- **Displacement (Elasticity)**
- **Velocity (Momentum; Damping)**
- **Acceleration**
- **What are the phasic relations?**

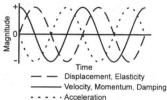

— — Displacement, Elasticity
——— Velocity, Momentum, Damping
- - - - · Acceleration

Ch2-61

Review of SHM and Important Phasic Relations

- **Learned previously that**
  - ◆ c leads x by 90°
  - ◆ a leads c by 90°, and
  - ◆ a leads x by 180°

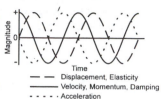

— — Displacement, Elasticity
——— Velocity, Momentum, Damping
- - - - · Acceleration

Ch2-62

Review of SHM and Important Phasic Relations

- **In addition**
  - ◆ E is in phase with x; Hooke's Law
  - ◆ M is in phase with c
  - ◆ Damping also in phase with c

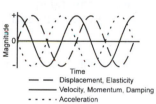

— — Displacement, Elasticity
——— Velocity, Momentum, Damping
- - - - · Acceleration

Ch2-63

Effects of Friction on Vibratory Motion

- **Friction limits velocity**
- **Amplitude of vibration diminishes over time**
- **Vibrations are damped**

Ch2-64

Effects of Friction on Vibratory Motion

- **In SHM, damping varies sinusoidally over time: it is <u>in phase with velocity</u>**
- **As velocity increases, kinetic energy is transformed to thermal energy: system is damped**

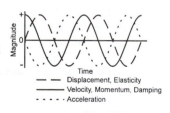

— — Displacement, Elasticity
——— Velocity, Momentum, Damping
- - - - · Acceleration

Ch2-65

The Magnitude of Damping

- **Magnitude of displacement depends on force applied**
- **Duration of vibration depends on magnitude of damping re: force applied**

Ch2-66

The Magnitude of Damping

- In Figure,
  - ◆ Panel A: lossless system
  - ◆ Panel B: low-damped system
  - ◆ Panel C: high-damped system

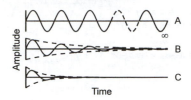

Ch2-67

The Damping Factor

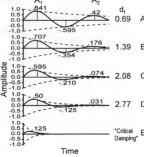

- Ratio of amplitudes of any two consecutive cycles is a constant
- $A_1 / A_2 = A_2 / A_3 = A_N / A_{N+1}$
- $d_f = \ln (A_1 / A_2)$
- From panels A-D, d_f increases from 0.69 to 2.77
- Panel E: critical damping

Ch2-68

Examples of Damped Systems

- Shock absorbers (nearly critically damped)

- VU meter (nearly critically damped)

- What would happen if they were nearly undamped?

  ☑

Ch2-69

ACOUSTIC IMPEDANCE

- System engages in SHM: it vibrates freely at its natural frequency (f_{nat})

- $f_{nat} = \sqrt{s/m}$

- What are the proportional relations of f_{nat} with s and m?

  ☑

  ☑

Ch2-70

ACOUSTIC IMPEDANCE

- Forces exist that oppose, or impede, motion: Impedance (Z)
- Total impedance has two components:
  - ◆ resistance   R
  - ◆ reactance   X
    - >> mass reactance X_m
    - >> compliant reactance X_c

Ch2-71

Resistance (R)

- Friction, or frictional resistance, occurs: kinetic energy is transformed to thermal energy

- Resistance measured in ohms (Ω)

- Resistance is independent of frequency!

Ch2-72

Reactance (X)

- Forces that oppose motion in a frequency selective way: <u>frequency dependent</u>

- With R, <u>energy is dissipated</u>

- With X, <u>energy is stored as PE</u>

Ch2-73

Two Components of Impedance

- 1. Energy-dissipating: What is it?
  ☑

- 2. Energy-storage: What is it?
  ☑

- Impedance: Complex sum of R & X

Ch2-74

Reactance

- Reactance depends on mass and compliance of the system

- Both mass and compliance oppose, or impede, motion

  - But in opposite ways

  - Can understand the difference by review of certain phasic relations

Ch2-75

Crucial Phasic Relations

- Opposition to motion from Resistance is <u>in phase</u> with <u>velocity</u>
  - Resistance: in phase with c, M, and damping

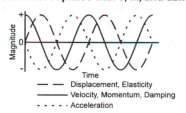

— — Displacement, Elasticity
——— Velocity, Momentum, Damping
- - - - · Acceleration

Ch2-76

Crucial Phasic Relations

- Opposition to motion from Compliance is <u>in phase</u> with <u>elasticity</u>; <u>lags</u> Resistance by 90°
  - Compliance: in phase with E and x

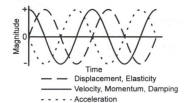

— — Displacement, Elasticity
——— Velocity, Momentum, Damping
- - - - · Acceleration

Ch2-77

Crucial Phasic Relations

- Opposition to motion from Mass is <u>in phase</u> with <u>acceleration</u>;
  - leads resistance by 90°
- Opposition to motion from <u>Mass</u> is 180° <u>out of phase</u> with opposition to motion from <u>Compliance</u>

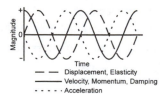

— — Displacement, Elasticity
——— Velocity, Momentum, Damping
- - - - · Acceleration

Ch2-78

Two Components of X: X_m and X_c

- When one reactance component stores energy, the other gives up energy

- They are 180° out of phase with one another

- They <u>act in opposition</u> to one another

Mass Reactance: X_m

- Also measured in ohms (Ω)
- $X_m = 2\pi fm$
- X_m is <u>directly proportional</u> to frequency
- Negligible at low frequencies
- For every octave (2:1) increase in f, X_m doubles
-

X_m vs f — line rising to the right

Mass Reactance: X_m

- At low frequencies,
  - ♦ X_m negligible; larger amplitude of vibration
- At high frequencies,
  - ♦ X_m large; smaller amplitude of vibration
- Can demonstrate with low-pass filter

Compliant Reactance: X_c

- Also measured in ohms (Ω)
- $X_c = 1/2\pi fc$
- X_c is <u>inversely proportional</u> to frequency
- Large at low frequencies
-

X_c vs f — curve decreasing to the right

Compliant Reactance: X_c

- At low frequencies,
  - ♦ X_c large; smaller amplitude of vibration
- At high frequencies,
  - ♦ X_c negligible; larger amplitude of vibration
- Can demonstrate with high-pass filter

Mass Reactance (X_m) and Compliant Reactance (X_c)

- What if $X_m = X_c$?
  - ♦ If $X_m = X_c$, X = 0
  - ♦ Z = R
  - ♦ Impedance is minimal
  - ♦ Amplitude of vibration is largest
  - ♦ f_{nat}

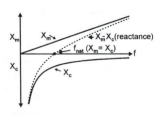

Mass Reactance (X_m) and Compliant Reactance (X_c)

- $f < f_{nat}$
  - ◆ Z increases
  - ◆ Amplitude of vibration decreases
  - ◆ Compliance dominant ($X_c = 1/2\pi fc$)

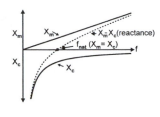

Ch2-85

Mass Reactance (X_m) and Compliant Reactance (X_c)

- $f > f_{nat}$
  - ◆ Z increases
  - ◆ Amplitude of vibration decreases
  - ◆ Mass dominant ($X_m = 2\pi fm$)

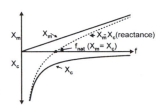

Ch2-86

Impedance (Z)

- R causes energy to be dissipated
- X causes energy to be stored as PE
  - ◆ X_m leads R by 90°
  - ◆ X_c lags R by 90°
  - ◆ X_m leads X_c by 180°

Ch2-87

Impedance

- $X_m = X_c$
- X_m, X_c, & R are vector-like quantities
- Called <u>phasor quantities</u>, or <u>phasors</u>
  - ◆ $Z = R$
  - ◆ f_{nat}

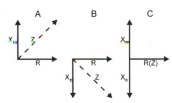

Ch2-88

Impedance

- Panel A: ($X_m > X_c$)
  - ◆ mass dominant
  - ◆ $Z > R$
- Panel B: ($X_m < X_c$)
  - ◆ compliance dominant
  - ◆ $Z > R$

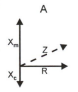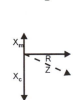

Ch2-89

Impedance

- $Z = \sqrt{R^2 + X_m{}^2}$
- $Z = \sqrt{R^2 + X_c{}^2}$
- $Z = \sqrt{R^2 + (X_m - X_c)^2}$

Ch2-90

Chapter 3

LOGARITHMS
AND ANTILOGARITHMS

THE CONCEPT OF LOGARITHMS AND ANTILOGARITHMS

- Sample problems
  - $\text{Antilog}_2 2 = ?$
  - $\text{Antilog}_2 3 = ?$
  - $\text{Antilog}_{10} 2 = ?$
  - $\text{Antilog}_{10} 3 = ?$
  - $2^2 = ?$ $2^3 = ?$
  - $10^2 = ?$ $10^3 = ?$

Sample Problems

- Equivalent problems

  - $\text{Antilog}_2 2 = 2^2 = 2 \times 2 = 4$

  - $\text{Antilog}_2 3 = 2^3 = 2 \times 2 \times 2 = 8$

  - $\text{Antilog}_{10} 2 = 10^2 = 10 \times 10 = 100$

  - $\text{Antilog}_{10} 3 = 10^3 = 10 \times 10 \times 10 = 1,000$

- Thus, $\text{antilog}_x n = x^n$

Sample Problems

- $\text{Antilog}_{10} 1.7 = ?$

  - Same concept

  - $10^{1.7} = ?$

  - Simply need to learn computational procedure

SCALES OF MEASUREMENT

- Distinction between numerals and numbers
- Numerals
  - Symbols that label
  - e.g., X, II, IX, 6, 9, etc.
  - 6 and 9, as <u>numerals</u>, <u>cannot</u> be added or subtracted

SCALES OF MEASUREMENT

- Numbers
  - Symbols with fixed relation to other symbols
  - 6 and 9, as <u>numbers</u>, <u>can</u> be added or subtracted

Four Scales of Measurement

- Nominal
- Ordinal
- Interval
- Ratio

Ch3-7

(1) Nominal Scale

- Objects are the <u>same</u> or <u>different</u>
- The <u>letter</u> A is different from the letter B
- The <u>numeral</u> 1 is different from the numeral 0
- Can sort into categories: Count the number of entries

Ch3-8

(2) Ordinal Scale

- Two things are the <u>same</u> or <u>different</u>, <u>and</u>
- One object has <u>more</u> or <u>less</u> of some quantity (or the same as) than another
- Thus:
  - ♦ A > B > C > D > F
  - ♦ F < D < C < B < A
  - ♦ 4 > 3 > 2 > 1 > 0

Ch3-9

Ordinal Scale

- Letters are <u>not</u> numbers: Cannot be added
- Numerals are <u>not</u> numbers either: Cannot be added

Ch3-10

Ordinal Scale

- Even if letters are replaced by numerals:

  - ♦ A = 4, B = 3, C = 2, D = 1, F = 0

  - ♦ The numerals still cannot be added

Ch3-11

Example

- Four men want to play a "competitive" golf match of doubles: Boomer (B), Draw (D), Slice (S), and Rake (R)
- Use driving range to establish rank order
  - ♦ B > D > S > R
- Assign numerals
  - ♦ B = 4, D = 3, S = 2, R = 1
  - ♦ 4 + 1 = 5; 3 + 2 = 5; So
  - ♦ B + R vs. D + S
  - ♦ D + S defeat B + R handily

Ch3-12

Example

- **What is the fallacy?**
  - ◆ Numerals were treated as numbers
  - ◆ B, D, and S were players of tournament quality
  - ◆ Rake tended the sand traps; had never swung a club before
- **The size of the interval between adjacent <u>numerals</u> was not known and was not a constant**

(3) Interval (Linear) Scale

- **Size of interval between adjacent <u>numbers</u> is known and is a constant**
- **Size of interval is called the BASE**
- **Successive units formed by adding (or subtracting) base to each number**

Interval Scale

- **Because BASE is known, we can say that one object is <u>a certain number of intervals more or less than another</u>**
  - ◆ Base = 1
    5 is 1 interval > 4
  - ◆ Base = 2
    6 is 1 interval < 8
  - ◆ Base = 10
    20 is 3 intervals < 50

Table 3-1. Examples of Interval Scales

Base	Scale	Interval Size
1	1, 2, 3, 4, 5, 6, ..., n	1
1	0, 1, 2, 3, 4, 5, ..., n	1
2	0, 2, 4, 6, 8, 10, ..., n	2
2	10, 8, 6, 4, 2, 0, ..., n	2
10	10, 20, 30, 40, 50, 60, ..., n	10

(4) Ratio (Exponential, or Logarithmic) Scale

- **One unit on scale is so many <u>times</u> greater or less than another**
- **Successive units formed by multiplying (or dividing) each number by the BASE**
- **Successive units differ by a <u>constant ratio</u>, which is the BASE**

Table 3-2. Examples of Ratio Scales

Base	Scale
1	1, 1, 1, 1, 1, ..., 1
2	1, 2, 4, 8, 16, 32, 64, ..., n
1.5	1, 1.5, 2.25, 3.375, 5.0625, ..., n
10	1, 10, 100, 1,000, 10,000, ..., n
0.1	1, .1, .01, .001, .0001, ..., n

Ratio Scale

- **Thus,**
  - ◆ Base = 2: 8 ÷ 4 = 2; 16 ÷ 8 = 2; etc.
  - ◆ Base = 10: 100 ÷ 10 = 10; 1,000 ÷ 100 = 10; etc.
  - ◆ Base = 1.5: 2.25 ÷ 1.5 = 1.5; 3.575 ÷ 2.25 = 1.5; etc.
  - ◆ Base = .1: .01 ÷ .1 = .1; .001 ÷ .01 = .1; etc.
- **If scale values are: 1, 3, 9, 27, and 81, What is the base?**
  - ☑
  - ☑

Ratio Scale

- **Why can a ratio scale be called an exponential scale?**
- **The scale of numbers can be represented as <u>the BASE raised to some power, or exponent</u>**

Examples

- Base = 2

  - $2^0 = 1$

  - $2^1 = 2$

  - $2^2 = 4$

  - $2^3 = 8$

  - $2^4 = 16$

Ch3-19

Ratio Scale

- **The numbers on the scale differ by a constant ratio, and**

- **They can be expressed as the base, 2 in this case, raised to progressively higher powers**

  - $2^0; 2^1; 2^2; 2^3; 2^4$

Ch3-20

Ratio Scale

- **Write a parallel scale where base = 3**

  - ☑
  - ☑
  - ☑
  - ☑
  - ☑

Ch3-21

Ratio Scale

- **Defining equation for exponential series:**

  - $X^n = \#$

- **That means the BASE $\underline{x}$ is to be used $\underline{n}$ times in multiplication**

Table 3-3. Base = 2 raised to powers of 3, 4, and 5

X^n	Operation	Result
2^3	$2 \times 2 \times 2$	8
2^4	$2 \times 2 \times 2 \times 2$	16
2^5	$2 \times 2 \times 2 \times 2 \times 2$	32

Ch3-22

Ratio Scale

Table 3-4. Exponential series for base = 2 and base = 10

Base = 2		Base = 10	
X^n	Result	X^n	Result
2^0	1	10^0	1
2^1	2	10^1	10
2^2	4	10^2	100
2^3	8	10^3	1,000
2^4	16	10^4	10,000
2^5	32	10^5	100,000

- **With either base, 2 or 10, successive entries on the scale that results differ by a <u>constant ratio</u>**

Ch3-23

Two Important Facts

- **Any BASE raised to the zero power (X^0) equals 1**

  - $X^0 = 1$

  - **Thus, $2^0 = 1$, $10^0 = 1$, $3^0 = 1$, etc**

- **Any BASE raised to the first power (X^1) equals the BASE**

  - $X^1 = X$

  - **Thus, $2^1 = 2$, $10^1 = 10$, $3^1 = 3$, etc**

Ch3-24

MORE ON EXPONENTS

- **Exponents specify how many times the BASE x is used in multiplication or division**
- **Multiplication**
  - $x^n = \#$
    - $\gg 5^4 = 5 \times 5 \times 5 \times 5 = 625$
    - $\gg 5^5 = 5 \times 5 \times 5 \times 5 \times 5 = 3125$
    - $\gg 2^4 = ?$
      - ☑

Ch3-25

MORE ON EXPONENTS

- **Division**
  - $x^{-n} = \#$
  - $x^{-n} = 1/x^n$
    - $\gg 2^{-2} = 1/2^2 = 1/4$
    - $\gg 10^{-4} = ?$
      - ☑

Ch3-26

Three Facts Restated

- $x^0 = 1$
- $x^1 = x$
- $x^{-n} = 1/x^n$
  - $5^{-4} = ?$
    - ☑

Ch3-27

Sample Problems

- $2^6 = ?$
  - ☑
  - ☑
- $10^6 = ?$
  - ☑
  - ☑
- $2^{-6} = ?$
  - ☑

Ch3-28

Sample Problems

- $10^{-6} = ?$
  - ☑
- $7.16^1 = ?$
  - ☑
- $7.16^0 = ?$
  - ☑

Ch3-29

Laws of Exponents

- **1) Law 1: $(x^a) \cdot (x^b) = x^{a+b}$**
  - $2^4 \times 2^2 = 2^{4+2} = 2^6 = 64$
  - $2^{1.4} \times 2^{3.6} = 2^{1.4+3.6} = 2^5 = 32$
- **The product of some base x raised to some power, and the same base x raised to the same or different power, equals the base raised to the sum of the two powers**

Ch3-30

Laws of Exponents

- 2) Law 2: $x^a/x^b = x^{a-b}$

  - $2^6/2^4 = 2^{6-4} = 2^2 = 4$

  - $2^{5.5}/2^{3.5} = 2^{5.5-3.5} = 2^2 = 4$

- The <u>ratio</u> of some base x raised to some power, to the same base raised to the same or different power, equals the base raised to the <u>difference</u> between the powers

  Ch3-31

Law 2

- **More examples**

  - $10^{-8}/10^{-13} = 10^5$

  - $10^{-13}/10^{-8} = 10^{-5}$

  - $10^{-7}/10^{-7} = 10^0 = 1$

- **Any number divided by itself must equal 1: Hence $10^0 = 1$ and, more generally, $x^0 = 1$**

  Ch3-32

Laws of Exponents

- 3) Law 3: $(x^a)^b = x^{ab}$

  - $(10^2)^3 = (10)^{2 \cdot 3} = 10^6$

  Ch3-33

LOGS AND ANTILOGS:
Antilogs

- Form two exponential series: Base = 2 and Base = 10
- We ask: $X^n = ?$

Table 3-5. Two exponential series of numbers for base = 2 and base = 10

Base = 2		Base = 10	
X^n	Answer	X^n	Answer
$2^0 = ?$	1	$10^0 = ?$	1
$2^1 = ?$	2	$10^1 = ?$	10
$2^2 = ?$	4	$10^2 = ?$	100
$2^3 = ?$	8	$10^3 = ?$	1,000
$2^4 = ?$	16	$10^4 = ?$	10,000

Ch3-34

Antilogs

- What is 2 raised to the 0, 1, 2, 3, or 4 power?

  or

- What is 10 raised to the 0, 1, 2, 3, or 4 power?
- GENERALLY: What is the value of the base X raised to the nth power? $X^n = ?$

Table 3-5. Two exponential series of numbers for base = 2 and base = 10

Base = 2		Base = 10	
X^n	Answer	X^n	Answer
$2^0 = ?$	1	$10^0 = ?$	1
$2^1 = ?$	2	$10^1 = ?$	10
$2^2 = ?$	4	$10^2 = ?$	100
$2^3 = ?$	8	$10^3 = ?$	1,000
$2^4 = ?$	16	$10^4 = ?$	10,000

Ch3-35

Antilogs

- That is the same as <u>determining the antilog of a number</u>
- Thus,

  - $X^n = ?$ is the same as $\text{antilog}_x n = ?$

  - $2^5 = 32$ and $\text{antilog}_2 5 = 32$

  - $10^3 = 1,000$ and $\text{antilog}_{10} 3 = 1,000$

Table 3-5. Two exponential series of numbers for base = 2 and base = 10

Base = 2		Base = 10	
X^n	Answer	X^n	Answer
$2^0 = ?$	1	$10^0 = ?$	1
$2^1 = ?$	2	$10^1 = ?$	10
$2^2 = ?$	4	$10^2 = ?$	100
$2^3 = ?$	8	$10^3 = ?$	1,000
$2^4 = ?$	16	$10^4 = ?$	10,000

Ch3-36

Sample Problems

- Antilog$_2$ 6 = ?
  ☑
- Antilog$_{10}$ 5 = ?
  ☑
- Antilog$_3$ 2 = ?
  ☑

Ch3-37

Sample Problems

- Antilog$_{10}$ -2 = ?
  ♦ $x^{-n} = 1/x^n$
  ♦ antilog$_x$ -n = 1/antilog$_x$ n
  ♦ $1/10^2 = .01$
- Antilog$_{10}$ 0 = ?
  ☑
- Antilog$_{10}$ 1 = ?
  ☑

Ch3-38

LOGS AND ANTILOGS:
Logs

- The exponent is not given
- We ask: To what power must the BASE be raised to equal some number?
  ♦ $x^? = \#$
  ♦ $2^? = 8$
  ♦ $10^? = 10,000$
- Solving for an exponent

Table 3-6. Two exponential series for base = 2 and base = 10

Base = 2		Base = 10	
X^n	Answer	X^n	Answer
$2^? = 1$	0	$10^? = 1$	0
$2^? = 2$	1	$10^? = 10$	1
$2^? = 4$	2	$10^? = 100$	2
$2^? = 8$	3	$10^? = 1,000$	3
$2^? = 16$	4	$10^? = 10,000$	4

Ch3-39

Taking the Log of a Number

- Log$_2$ 8 = 3
  $2^? = 8$
- Log$_{10}$ 10,000 = 4
  $10^? = 10,000$
- Log$_{10}$ 1,000,000 = 6
  $10^? = 1,000,000$

Table 3-6. Two exponential series for base = 2 and base = 10

Base = 2		Base = 10	
X^n	Answer	X^n	Answer
$2^? = 1$	0	$10^? = 1$	0
$2^? = 2$	1	$10^? = 10$	1
$2^? = 4$	2	$10^? = 100$	2
$2^? = 8$	3	$10^? = 1,000$	3
$2^? = 16$	4	$10^? = 10,000$	4

Ch3-40

Taking the Log of a Number

	Ratio Scale	Linear Scale
● Log$_{10}$ 10,000 =		4
	10:1	
● Log$_{10}$ 1,000 =		3
	10:1	
● Log$_{10}$ 100 =		2
	10:1	
● Log$_{10}$ 10 =		1
	10:1	
● Log$_{10}$ 1 =		0

Ch3-41

Taking the Log of a Number

	Between	Thus
● Log$_{10}$ 200 =	2 & 3	2.xx
● Log$_{10}$ 700 =	2 & 3	2.xx
● Log$_{10}$ 3,000 =	3 & 4	3.xx
● Log$_{10}$ 27 =	1 & 2	1.xx
● Log$_{10}$ 5 =	0 & 1	0.xx
● Log$_{10}$ 0.5=	0 & -1	?

  ♦ We will see answer later

Ch3-42

Bases for Logs and Antilogs

- The BASE <u>must be specified</u>
- Any number (other than 1) can be the BASE
- Three BASES are ordinarily encountered
  - ♦ 2
  - ♦ 10 (Common or Briggsian Log)
  - ♦ e (2.718: Natural or Naperian Log)

Ch3-43

Summary

- When you take the <u>log</u> of a number, you are solving for an <u>exponent</u>
  - ♦ An <u>exponent</u> is a <u>log</u>
  - ♦ A <u>log</u> is an <u>exponent</u>

Ch3-44

PROCEDURES FOR SOLVING LOG AND ANTILOG PROBLEMS:
Logs

- $\text{Log}_{10}\ 100 = ?$ Obvious
  - ☑
- $\text{Log}_{10}\ 1{,}000 = ?$ Obvious
  - ☑
- $\text{Log}_{10}\ 150 = ?$ Not so obvious
  - ☑
  - ☑

Ch3-45

Components (Anatomy) of a Log

Integer Decimal Values

- $\text{Log}_{10}\ 100 = 2.000000000$
- $\text{Log}_{10}\ 1{,}000 = 3.000000000$
- $\text{Log}_{10}\ 150 = 2.176091259$

Ch3-46

Components of a Log

- Integer: the <u>characteristic</u>
- Decimals: the <u>mantissa</u>
  - ♦ $\text{Log}_{10}\ 150 = 2.176091259$
  - ♦ Characteristic = 2.
  - ♦ Mantissa   = .176091259

Ch3-47

How to Solve Log Problems

- Calculator
- Log table
  - ♦ If log table, it is helpful to convert <u>conventional number</u> into <u>scientific notation</u>
  - ♦ Scientific notation, however, is important in its own right

Ch3-48

Scientific Notation

- A number written in scientific notation is expressed as the product of a coefficient and the base 10 raised to some power
- The coefficient
  - ♦ A number equal to or greater than 1.00, but
  - ♦ less than 10 (e.g., 1.0000; 3.14159; 9.9999)
- See Table 3-7

Ch3-49

Scientific Notation

Table 3-7. Comparison of conventional and scientific notation

Conventional Notation	Scientific Notation
10	1.00×10^1
100	1.00×10^2
1,000	1.00×10^3
121	1.21×10^2
800	8.00×10^2
0.1	1.00×10^{-1}
0.0121	1.21×10^{-2}

Ch3-50

Procedure

- Move decimal point leftward (successive division by 10) or rightward (successive multiplication by 10) until requirements for <u>coefficient</u> are met
- The number of places moved specifies the <u>value</u> of the exponent
  - ♦ Successive division: + exponent
  - ♦ Successive multiplication: − exponent

Ch3-51

Examples

- $100 = 1.00 \times 10^2$
- $200 = 2.00 \times 10^2$
- $300 = 3.00 \times 10^2$
- $315 = 3.15 \times 10^2$

- 0.125 = ?
  - ☑
- 0.0367 = ?
  - ☑
- 0.000001 = ?
  - ☑

Ch3-52

Examples

- $100 = 10^2$ (or) 1×10^2
- $1,000 = 10^3$ (or) 1×10^3
- $200 = ?$
  - ☑
- $2,000 = ?$
  - ☑

Ch3-53

Scientific Notation

- A number, in scientific notation, is the product of some simple number (the <u>coefficient</u>) and 10 raised to some <u>power</u>
- 12500 = ?
  - ☑
- 12541 = ?
  - ☑

Ch3-54

Scientific Notation

- **When the number, in conventional notation, is 10 or greater:**

  - **Count the number of places that the decimal point must be moved to the <u>left</u> to lie between 1 and 9 (successive division by 10)**

- **This specifies the <u>positive</u> exponent**

  - $114 = 1.14 \times 10^2$

Ch3-55

Scientific Notation

- **When the number, in conventional notation, is less than 1:**

  - **Count the number of places that the decimal point must be moved to the <u>right</u> (successive multiplication by 10)**

- **This specifies the <u>negative</u> exponent**

  - $.114 = 1.14 \times 10^{-1}$

Ch3-56

Scientific Notation

- **When the number, in conventional notation, equals 1:**

  - **The decimal point need not be moved**

- **The exponent is <u>zero</u>**

  - $1.00 = 1.00 \times 10^0$

  - $9.00 = 9.00 \times 10^0$

Ch3-57

Solution For Logs

- **Three steps for solution of log problems: $Log_{10}\ 145 = ?$**

- **Step 1: Express number in scientific notation**

  - $Log_{10}\ 145 = log_{10}\ 1.45 \times 10^2$

- **Step 2: The <u>exponent</u> in scientific notation is the <u>characteristic</u> of the log**

  - $Log_{10}\ 1.45 \times 10^2 = 2.xxxx$

Ch3-58

Solution For Logs

- **Step 3: Look up <u>mantissa</u> in a log table**

  - **The first two digits of coefficient indicate proper <u>row</u> in log table; the third digit specifies the correct <u>column</u>. Thus, 1.45 directs you to row 14 and column 5**

  - $Log_{10}\ 1.45 \times 10^2 = 2.1614$

Ch3-59

Log Table

N	0	1	2	3	4	5	6	7	8	9
10	0.0000	0.0043	0.0086	0.0128	0.0170	0.0212	0.0253	0.0294	0.0334	0.0374
11	0.0414	0.0453	0.0492	0.0531	0.0569	0.0607	0.0645	0.0682	0.0719	0.0755
12	0.0792	0.0828	0.0864	0.0899	0.0934	0.0969	0.1004	0.1038	0.1072	0.1106
13	0.1139	0.1173	0.1206	0.1239	0.1271	0.1303	0.1335	0.1367	0.1399	0.1430
14	0.1461	0.1492	0.1523	0.1553	0.1584	0.1614	0.1644	0.1673	0.1703	0.1732
15	0.1761	0.1790	0.1818	0.1847	0.1875	0.1903	0.1931	0.1959	0.1987	0.2014
16	0.2041	0.2068	0.2095	0.2122	0.2148	0.2175	0.2201	0.2227	0.2253	0.2279
17	0.2304	0.2330	0.2355	0.2380	0.2405	0.2430	0.2455	0.2480	0.2504	0.2529
18	0.2553	0.2577	0.2601	0.2625	0.2648	0.2672	0.2695	0.2718	0.2742	0.2765
19	0.2788	0.2810	0.2833	0.2856	0.2878	0.2900	0.2923	0.2945	0.2967	0.2989
20	0.3010	0.3032	0.3054	0.3075	0.3096	0.3118	0.3139	0.3160	0.3181	0.3201
21	0.3222	0.3243	0.3263	0.3284	0.3304	0.3324	0.3345	0.3365	0.3385	0.3404
22	0.3424	0.3444	0.3464	0.3483	0.3502	0.3522	0.3541	0.3560	0.3579	0.3598
23	0.3617	0.3636	0.3655	0.3674	0.3692	0.3711	0.3729	0.3747	0.3766	0.3784
24	0.3802	0.3820	0.3838	0.3856	0.3874	0.3892	0.3909	0.3927	0.3945	0.3962
25	0.3979	0.3997	0.4014	0.4031	0.4048	0.4065	0.4082	0.4099	0.4116	0.4133
26	0.4150	0.4166	0.4183	0.4200	0.4216	0.4232	0.4249	0.4265	0.4281	0.4298
27	0.4314	0.4330	0.4346	0.4362	0.4378	0.4393	0.4409	0.4425	0.4440	0.4456
28	0.4472	0.4487	0.4502	0.4518	0.4533	0.4548	0.4564	0.4579	0.4594	0.4609
29	0.4624	0.4639	0.4654	0.4669	0.4683	0.4698	0.4713	0.4728	0.4742	0.4757

Ch3-60

Sample Problems

- Log_{10} 846 =
  ☑
- Log_{10} 923 =
  ☑
- Log_{10} 1,000 =
  ☑

Ch3-61

Sample Problems

- Log_{10} 2,315 =
  ☑
- Log_{10} 1 =
  ☑
- NOTE: If $x^0 = 1$, and if an exponent is a log, then the Log_{10} 1 = 0 !

Ch3-62

Sample Problems

- Log_{10} 2 =
  ☑
- Log_{10} 0.0002 =
  ☑
- NOTE: The characteristic can be positive <u>or</u> negative, but the mantissa can <u>only</u> be positive

Ch3-63

Explanation

- Log 2000   • 3.3
- Log 1000   • 3
- Log 200   • 2.3
- Log 100   • 2
- Log 20   • 1.3
- Log 10   • 1
- Log 2   • 0.3
- Log 1   • 0

- Note: Each bracket spans one power of 10 and represents 1 log unit because log_{10} 10 = 1

Ch3-64

Explanation

- Log .2   • -1.3? NO! $\overline{1}.3$ = - 0.7
- Log .1   • $\overline{1}$
- Log .02   • $\overline{2}.3$
- Log .01   • $\overline{2}$
- Log .002   • $\overline{3}.3$
- Log .001   • $\overline{3}$
- Log .0002   • $\overline{4}.3$
- Log .0001   • $\overline{4}$

- .2 is one power of 10 <u>less</u> than 2 and therefore is 1 log unit <u>less</u> than the log of 2
  ♦ 0.3 - 1 = - 0.7

Ch3-65

Logs With Bases Other Than 10

- $log_Y X = log_{10} X / log_{10} Y$

  ♦ $log_2 8 = log_{10} 8 / log_{10} 2$

  ♦   = .9031 / .3010

  ♦   = 3

Ch3-66

PROCEDURES FOR SOLVING LOG AND ANTILOG PROBLEMS:
Antilogs

- Same three steps used for solving log problems, but in reverse order
  - ◆ Antilog$_{10}$ 2.1614 (>100; <1,000)
- Step 1

  .1614 is the <u>mantissa</u>. Find 1614 as cell entry in log table. The two-digit row and one-digit column designators yield the <u>coefficient</u> in scientific notation: 1.45
  - ◆ Antilog$_{10}$ 2.1614 = 1.45 × 10$^?$

Ch3-67

Solutions For Antilogs

- Step 2:

  The characteristic is 2. It yields the <u>exponent</u> in scientific notation.
  - ◆ Therefore: Antilog$_{10}$ 2.1614 = 1.45 × 10^2 = 145

Ch3-68

Logs and Antilogs with a Calculator

- Logs: Log$_{10}$ 167 = ?
  - ◆ Enter # in key pad: 167
  - ◆ Press log key
  - ◆ Display shows 2.2227
- Antilogs: Antilog$_{10}$ 2.2227
  - ◆ Enter # in key pad: 2.2227
  - ◆ Press 10^x key
  - ◆ Display shows 167

Ch3-69

Laws of Logarithms

- 1. Law 1: Log ab = Log a + Log b
  - ◆ Log (10 × 10) = ?
  - ◆ Log 10 + Log 10 = 2
- You have encountered this law before: when a conventional number is expressed in scientific notation, you find the log of the product of a coefficient and 10^x by summing the log of the coefficient and the log of 10^x

Ch3-70

Law 1

- Log 145 = ?
  - ◆ Log (1.45 × 10^2) =
  - ◆ Log 1.45 + Log 10^2 =
  - ◆ 2 + .1614 = 2.1614

Ch3-71

Laws of Logarithms

- 2. Law 2: Log a/b = Log a - Log b
  - ◆ Log (100/10) = ?
  - ◆ Log 100 - Log 10 =
  - ◆ 2 - 1 = 1
- Law 2 will be encountered repeatedly in solution of decibel problems

Ch3-72

Law 2

- Log (2.16 / 1.58) = ?
  - ◆ Log 2.16 - Log 1.58 =
  - ◆ 0.3345 - 0.1987 =
  - ◆ 0.1358
- Log $(1 \times 10^4) / (2 \times 10^2)$ = ?
  - ◆ Log 10^4 - Log (2×10^2) =
  - ◆ 4 - 2.3 = 1.7
  - ◆ Note: in this problem we applied both Law 1 and Law 2

Ch3-73

Laws of Logarithms

- 3. Law 3: Log a^b = b Log a
  - ◆ Log 10^2 = 2 Log 10 = 2×1 = 2
  - ◆ Log 10^3 = 3 Log 10 = 3×1 = 3
  - ◆ Log $10^{2.75}$ = 2.75 Log 10 = 2.75
  - ◆ Log $6^{3.5}$ = 3.5 Log 6 = $3.5 \times .78$
    = 2.72
- This law will be used to derive the equation for decibels for <u>pressure</u> from the equation for decibels for <u>intensity</u> in Chapter 4

Ch3-74

Laws of Logarithms

- 4. Law 4: Log 1 / a = - Log a
  - ◆ Log (1 / 10) = - Log 10 = - 1
  - ◆ Log (1 / 12) = - Log 12 = - 1.08
- This law will be encountered in solving problems in Chapters 5 and 8

Ch3-75

Logs Without Log Tables or Calculators

- Log 1 = 0
- Log 2 = .3
- Log 3 = .48
- Log 4 =
  - ☑
- Log 5 =
  - ☑
- Log 6 =
  - ☑

- MEMORIZE
- MEMORIZE
- MEMORIZE

Ch3-76

Logs Without Log Tables or Calculators

- Log 7 = .85
- Log 8 =
  - ☑
- Log 9 =
  - ☑
- Log 10 =
  - ☑

- MEMORIZE

Ch3-77

Chapter 4

SOUND INTENSITY AND SOUND PRESSURE: THE DECIBEL

Ch4-1

Acoustic Power

- Sound energy is transferred through a medium at some rate
- POWER: The rate at which energy is transferred; Energy transferred per unit time
- ENERGY: The capacity to do work, whereas POWER is the rate at which energy is expended

Ch4-2

Unit of Measure

- The WATT

  ◆ 1 Watt = 1 joule/s (MKS): a force of 1 newton acting through a distance of 1 meter = 1 joule

  Or

  ◆ 10,000,000 (10^7) ergs/s (cgs): a force of 1 dyne acting through a distance of 1 centimeter = 1 erg

Ch4-3

ABSOLUTE AND RELATIVE MEASURES OF ACOUSTIC POWER

- Consider absolute and relative measures of height

  ◆ Building A is twice as tall as building B: A <u>relative</u> measure. You do not know the heights of A or B, but you know that A = 2B and B = A/2

  ◆ The height of A is 8 m and the height of B is 4 m: <u>absolute</u> measures

  ◆ From that knowledge, we can derive a relative measure: A = 2B and B = A/2

Ch4-4

Absolute Measure of Power

- Power is expressed in watts

  ◆ e. g., 60, 90, 150 watts (electricity)

  ◆ 2×10^{-8} watts (sound)

- The rate at which energy is consumed

Ch4-5

Relative Measure of Power

- Absolute power in one sound wave is compared with absolute power in another (<u>reference</u>) wave

  ◆ A = 2B, or B = A/2

  ◆ A = 10B, or B = A/10

    >> If A = 5×10^{-6}, then B = 5×10^{-7}

Ch4-6

Summary

- Level = W_x / W_r, where W_x is the power of interest and W_r is a reference power
- Light bulbs
  - ◆ 60 / 30 = 2
  - ◆ 100 / 30 = 3.33
  - ◆ 100 / 60 = 1.67
- A <u>ratio</u> of x to r

Ch4-7

Importance of Specifying the Reference Power

- The measure of level is <u>meaningless</u> unless W_r is specified
  - ◆ Level = 1,000 ?
  - ◆ Level = 1,000 re: 10^{-4} watt
  - >> You know that W_x is 1,000 (10^3) times greater than W_r and, because W_r is specified, you can calculate the value of W_x to be 10^{-1}

Ch4-8

SOUND INTENSITY

- An idealized point source of sound located in a free, unbounded medium
- Energy transferred from point source as an <u>ever-expanding</u> sphere (soap bubble analogy)
- We measure power dissipated (not over entire surface of sphere) on some <u>small area</u> (the <u>square meter</u> or <u>square centimeter</u>)

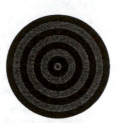

Ch4-9

SOUND INTENSITY

- Power: Energy per second
- Intensity: Energy per second per square meter (MKS)
- Units of Measure
  - ◆ Power: watt
  - ◆ Intensity: watt / m^2
  - ◆ What is unit in cgs system?
    ☑

Ch4-10

ABSOLUTE AND RELATIVE MEASURES OF SOUND INTENSITY

- Absolute: The intensity is:
  3.15×10^{-2} watt / m^2
- Relative: Level = I_x / I_r
  - ◆ A = 10B or B = A / 10

Ch4-11

Ratios I_x / I_r

- For each value of I_x, the ratio I_x / I_r (the <u>level</u>) depends on the value of I_r
- If $I_x = 10^{-10}$ watt / m^2, the level is:
  - ◆ 10^0 when $I_r = 10^{-10}$, but
  - ◆ 10^2 when $I_r = 10^{-12}$

Table 4-1. Ratios I_x / I_r for two different reference intensities

Absolute Intensity in watt/m^2 I_x	Relative Intensity, I_x / I_r, in watt/m^2	
	$I_r = 10^{-10}$	$I_r = 10^{-12}$
10^{-8}	10^2	10^4
10^{-9}	10^1	10^3
10^{-10}	10^0	10^2
10^{-11}	10^{-1}	10^1
10^{-12}	10^{-2}	10^0
10^{-13}	10^{-3}	10^{-1}

Ch4-12

Ratios I_x / I_r

- Note: you are using **Law 2 of exponents**
  - $10^{-10} / 10^{-10} = 10^0$
  - $10^{-10} / 10^{-12} = 10^2$

Table 4-1. Ratios I_x / I_r for two different reference intensities

Absolute Intensity in watt/m^2 I_x	Relative Intensity, I_x / I_r, in watt/m^2	
	$I_r = 10^{-10}$	$I_r = 10^{-12}$
10^{-8}	10^2	10^4
10^{-9}	10^1	10^3
10^{-10}	10^0	10^2
10^{-11}	10^{-1}	10^1
10^{-12}	10^{-2}	10^0
10^{-13}	10^{-3}	10^{-1}

Ch4-13

Ratios I_x / I_r

- It is meaningless to say, the level of intensity is, e.g., 10^2
  - $10^2 = 10^{-8} / 10^{-10}$ and
  - $10^2 = 10^{-10} / 10^{-12}$

Table 4-1. Ratios I_x / I_r for two different reference intensities

Absolute Intensity in watt/m^2 I_x	Relative Intensity, I_x / I_r, in watt/m^2	
	$I_r = 10^{-10}$	$I_r = 10^{-12}$
10^{-8}	10^2	10^4
10^{-9}	10^1	10^3
10^{-10}	10^0	10^2
10^{-11}	10^{-1}	10^1
10^{-12}	10^{-2}	10^0
10^{-13}	10^{-3}	10^{-1}

Ch4-14

THE DECIBEL

- Consider the following examples of <u>the level of intensity</u> (a ratio)
  - 1,000
  - 10,000,000
  - 0.001
  - 0.0000001
- The numbers are unnecessarily cumbersome

Ch4-15

THE DECIBEL

- To begin simplification, we rewrite them in scientific notation
  - $1,000 = 10^3$
  - $10,000,000 = 10^7$
  - $0.001 = 10^{-3}$
  - $0.0000001 = 10^{-7}$
- Then we can simplify further

Ch4-16

The Base and the Exponent

- <u>The base is redundant</u>: It is always 10: $10^3, 10^7, 10^{-3}, 10^{-7}$,
- Why not just record the exponents?
  - 3, 7, - 3, and - 7
- <u>An exponent is a log</u>
- Thus, when we record the exponent, <u>we have taken the log</u> of the number
- Level = $\log_{10} (I_x / I_r)$

Ch4-17

The Bel

- The log of the ratio I_x / I_r is called a <u>bel</u>
- N (bels) = $\log_{10} (I_x / I_r)$
- If the base is not specified in some subsequent equations and problems, assume base = 10

Ch4-18

The Bel

- For the previous four levels, we say the levels are:
  - ◆ 3 bels, 7 bels, - 3 bels, and - 7 bels
- What do positive (+) bels mean?
  - ☑
- What do negative (-) bels mean?
  - ☑

Ch4-19

Ratios I_x/I_r

- When $I_r = 10^{-10}$ watt/m^2, we express the levels of intensity as 2, 1, 0, -1, - 2, and - 3 bels
- When $I_r = 10^{-12}$ watt/m^2, we express the levels of intensity as 4, 3, 2, 1, 0, and -1 bels

Table 4-1. Ratios I_x / I_r for two different reference intensities

Absolute Intensity in watt/m^2 I_x	Relative Intensity, I_x / I_r, in watt/m^2	
	$I_r = 10^{-10}$	$I_r = 10^{-12}$
10^{-8}	10^2	10^4
10^{-9}	10^1	10^3
10^{-10}	10^0	10^2
10^{-11}	10^{-1}	10^1
10^{-12}	10^{-2}	10^0
10^{-13}	10^{-3}	10^{-1}

Ch4-20

Summary

- Set $I_x = 10^{-6}$ watt/m^2, and
- Set $I_r = 10^{-10}$ watt/m^2
- What is the absolute intensity, I_x?
  - ☑
- What is the level of intensity in bels?
  - ☑

Ch4-21

From the Bel to the Decibel

- Set $I_x = 2 \times 10^{-8}$ watt/m^2, and
- Set $I_r = 10^{-12}$ watt/m^2
- N bels $= \log_{10} (2 \times 10^{-8} / 10^{-12})$

$$= \log_{10} (2 \times 10^4)$$

$$= 4.3$$

Ch4-22

From the Bel to the Decibel

- A centimeter is 1/100 of a meter
  - ◆ Therefore, to convert from meters to centimeters, multiply by 100
  - ◆ 2 m = 200 cm
- Similarly, a <u>decibel</u> is 1/10 of a <u>bel</u>
  - ◆ Therefore, to convert from <u>bels</u> to <u>decibels</u>, multiply by 10
  - ◆ 4.3 bels = 43 decibels

Ch4-23

From the Bel to the Decibel

- N bels $= \log_{10} (I_x / I_r)$
- N dB $= 10 \log_{10} (I_x / I_r)$
- A decibel is 10 times the log of an intensity ratio or of a power ratio

Ch4-24

Grammar

- Singular: decibel & dB

- Plural: decibels & dB (not dBs)

Ch4-25

Sample Problems

- If $I_r = 10^{-12}$ watt/m^2
  - $I_x = 10^{-10}$:   dB = ? ☑
    $I_x = 10^{-9}$:   dB = ? ☑
    $I_x = 10^{-8}$:   dB = ? ☑
    $I_x = 10^{-6}$:   dB = ? ☑
    $I_x = 2 \times 10^{-6}$:   dB = ? ☑
    $I_x = 4 \times 10^{-6}$:   dB = ? ☑
    $I_x = 10^{-12}$:   dB = ? ☑
    $I_x = 10^{-13}$:   dB = ? ☑
    $I_x = 2 \times 10^{-13}$: dB = ? ☑   ☑

Ch4-26

What Have We Learned?

- For every 10 - fold change in I_x, dB changes by?

  ☑

- Why?

  ☑

Ch4-27

What Have We Learned?

- For every 2 - fold change in I_x, dB changes by?

  ☑

- Why?

  ☑

Ch4-28

What Have We Learned?

- What do 0 decibels mean?

  ☑

- What do positive decibels mean?

  ☑

- What do negative decibels mean?

  ☑

- You should now be prepared to solve Practice Problems -- Set 1 and Set 2

Ch4-29

Intensity Level (dB IL)

- <u>The reference intensity must always be specified</u>

- Standard reference intensity for dB IL:

  - MKS: $I_r = 10^{-12}$ watt/m^2

  - cgs: $I_r = 10^{-16}$ watt/cm^2

- When I_r has above values, and no other values, the decibel is called <u>decibels intensity level (dB IL)</u>

Ch4-30

Intensity Level (dB IL)

I_x (watt / m^2)	dB IL = ?
$I_x = 10^{-5}$:	☑
$I_x = 10^{-6}$:	☑
$I_x = 10^{-7}$:	☑
$I_x = 10^{-8}$:	☑
$I_x = 10^{-9}$:	☑
$I_x = 10^{-10}$:	☑
$I_x = 10^{-11}$:	☑
$I_x = 10^{-12}$:	☑
$I_x = 10^{-13}$:	☑
$I_x = 10^{-14}$:	☑

Ch4-31

Sample Problems

- Two steps to follow for solution of decibel problems

  - 1) Select proper equation (So far, you only have one to choose from)

  - 2) Form ratio, calculate log of the ratio, and multiply by 10

Ch4-32

Sample Problems

- Intensity increases by 2:1. How many dB?
  ☑
- Intensity increases by 10:1. How many dB?
  ☑
- $I_x = 10^{-5}$ watt / m^2. What is dB IL?
  ☑
- $I_x = 2 \times 10^{-5}$ watt / m^2. What is dB IL?
  ☑
- $I_x = 4 \times 10^{-5}$ watt / m^2. What is dB IL?
  ☑

Ch4-33

Sample Problems

- 3 dB corresponds to what <u>intensity ratio</u>?
  ☑
  ☑
  ☑
- You are given decibels and are solving for X, so the procedures are the reverse of those used to solve for decibels when given X
  - Divide decibels by 10, which gives you a logarithm (3 ÷ 10 = .3)
  - Then, antilog$_{10}$ .3 = 2

Ch4-34

Sample Problems

- 23 dB corresponds to what <u>intensity ratio</u>?
  - 23 = 10 log X = 200:1

    >> 2.3 = log X

    >> antilog$_{10}$ 2.3 = 2×10^2

Ch4-35

Sample Problems

- 24 dB corresponds to what <u>intensity ratio</u>?
  ☑
- 65 dB IL corresponds to what <u>intensity</u> (I_x)?
  ☑
  ☑
  ☑
  ☑
  ☑

Ch4-36

More Sample Problems

- If $I_x = 10^{-9}$ watt/m^2, dB IL = ?
  - ☑
- If $I_x = 2 \times 10^{-9}$ watt/m^2, dB IL = ?
  - ☑
  - ♦ What is simplest solution?
    - ☑
    - ☑

Ch4-37

Calculate dB for each Ratio

● Ratio	dB = ?
2:1	☑
10:1	☑
20:1	☑
40:1	☑
200:1	☑
400:1	☑

Ch4-38

Calculate dB for each Ratio

● Ratio	dB = ?
1:2	☑
1:10	☑
1:20	☑
$10^4 / 10^2$	☑
$10^2 / 10^4$	☑
$10^6 / 10^2$	☑

Ch4-39

Calculate dB for each Ratio

● Ratio	dB = ?
$10^{-9} / 10^{-12}$	☑
$2 \times 10^{-9} / 10^{-12}$	☑
$4 \times 10^{-9} / 10^{-12}$	☑
$8 \times 10^{-9} / 10^{-12}$	☑
$0.5 \times 10^{-9} / 10^{-12}$	☑

Ch4-40

Given dB, Calculate Intensity Ratio

- dB = 3
  - ☑
- dB = 6
  - ☑
- dB = 10
  - ☑
- dB = 13
  - ☑
  - ☑

Ch4-41

Given dB, Calculate Intensity Ratio

- dB = 20
  - ☑
- dB = 23
  - ☑
- dB = 26
  - ☑
- dB = 76
  - ☑
- dB = - 3
  - ☑
  - ☑

Ch4-42

Given dB IL, Calculate I_x re: 10^{-12} watt/m²

- dB IL = 20

    $20 = 10 \log (I_x / 10^{-12})$

    $2 = \log (I_x / 10^{-12})$

    $I_x = 10^2 \times 10^{-12}$

    $= 10^{-10}$

Given dB IL, Calculate I_x re: 10^{-12} watt/m²

- dB IL = 23
    - ☑
    - ☑

Given dB IL, Calculate I_x re: 10^{-12} watt/m²

- dB IL = 40
    - ☑
- dB IL = 46
    - ☑
- dB IL = 65
    - ☑
- You should now be prepared to solve Practice Problems -- Set 3 and Set 4

Summary Four Types of Problems

- 1. Given an intensity ratio, calculate decibels (Set 1)
- 2. Given decibels, calculate intensity ratio (Set 2)
- 3. Given I_x, calculate dB IL (Set 3)
- 4. Given dB IL, calculate I_x (Set 4)

SOUND PRESSURE

- Pressure is force/unit area
- Unit of measure (MKS):
    - ♦ N/m²
    - ♦ Pa, where 1 Pa = 1 N/m²
    - ♦ μN/m²
    - ♦ μPa, where
      1 μPa = 1 μN/m²

SOUND PRESSURE

- ♦ Note: In the cgs system, the unit is either the dyne/cm² or the microbar
- If p_x = 300 μPa (3×10^2), we refer to the <u>absolute pressure</u>
- To express in decibels, we <u>cannot</u> use the "10 log equation"
- To derive an appropriate equation, we will consider <u>intensity</u> and <u>pressure</u> in relation to impedance (Z)

Impedance

- Impedance (Z) can be described as the <u>product</u> of the <u>density</u> of a medium and the <u>speed</u> of wave propagation through the medium

  ♦ $Z_c = \rho_o s$

Impedance

- Intensity was defined previously as energy/s/m²

- Intensity also can be defined as the <u>ratio of rms pressure squared to the impedance</u>

  ♦ $I = p_{rms}^2 / Z_c$

  ♦ Thus: $I \propto p^2$

Decibels for Sound Pressure

- I is proportional to the square of rms pressure,
  ♦ $I \propto p^2$ (Remember!)
  ♦ and conversely
- rms pressure is proportional to the square root of I
  ♦ $p \propto \sqrt{I}$ (Remember!)
- $I = p^2 / Z_c$

Decibels for Sound Pressure

- Thus, if I increases by some factor, p <u>increases by the square root</u> of that factor: $p \propto \sqrt{I}$

  Or

- As rms pressure increases by some factor, I <u>increases by the square</u> of that factor: $I \propto p^2$

Decibels for Sound Pressure

- We cannot use the "10 log equation" for <u>pressure</u>, but we can derive one:
- $dB = 10 \log_{10} (I_x / I_r)$

  $= 10 \log_{10} (p_x^2 / Z) / (p_r^2 / Z)$

  $= 10 \log_{10} (p_x^2) / (p_r^2)$

  $= 10 \log_{10} (p_x / p_r)^2$

  $= 10 \times 2 \log_{10} (p_x / p_r)$ (Why?)

  ☑

  $= 20 \log_{10} (p_x / p_r)$

Decibels for Sound Pressure

- Thus, a decibel is 10 times the log of an <u>intensity</u> or <u>power</u> ratio

  ♦ $dB = 10 \log_{10} (I_x / I_r)$, and

- 20 times the log of a <u>pressure</u> ratio

  ♦ $dB = 20 \log_{10} (p_x / p_r)$

Sound Pressure Level: dB SPL

- dB IL: $I_r = 10^{-12}$ watt/m^2

- An intensity of 10^{-12} watt/m^2 creates a pressure in air of 20 (2×10^1) µPa

- Therefore, for dB SPL, the reference pressure, p_r, is 20 µPa

- $p_r = 2 \times 10^1$ µPa

Ch4-55

The Relation Between Absolute Pressure and Decibels

p_x (µ Pa)		dB SPL = ?
2×10^6	=	100

- ◆ dB SPL = $20 \log_{10} (2 \times 10^6 / 2 \times 10^1) = 100$

2×10^5	=	☑
2×10^4	=	☑
2×10^3	=	☑
2×10^2	=	☑
2×10^1	=	☑
2×10^0	=	☑
2×10^{-1}	=	☑

Ch4-56

Sample Problems

- Select the proper equation

    ◆ 10 log for intensity, or

    ◆ 20 log for pressure

- Form ratio and solve equation

Ch4-57

Sample Problems

- Pressure increases by 2:1. dB =
    ☑
- Pressure increases by 10:1. dB =
    ☑
- $p_x = 2 \times 10^5$ µPa. dB SPL =
    ☑
- $p_x = 4 \times 10^5$ µPa. dB SPL =
    ☑

    ◆ What is simplest solution?
        ☑

Ch4-58

Sample Problems

- $p_x = 8 \times 10^5$ µPa.
    ☑
    ◆ How did you solve it?
- 6 dB corresponds to what pressure ratio?
    ☑
- 26 dB corresponds to what pressure ratio?
    ☑

Ch4-59

Sample Problems

- 41 dB corresponds to what <u>pressure ratio</u>?

    ☑

Ch4-60

Sample Problems

- 60 dB SPL corresponds to what <u>absolute pressure</u>?

  ☑

1) Calculate dB for each Pressure Ratio

- 2:1
  ☑
- 10:1
  ☑
- 20:1
  ☑
- 40:1
  ☑
- 200:1
  ☑
- 400:1
  ☑

1) Calculate dB for each Pressure Ratio

- 1:2
  ☑
- 1:10
  ☑
- 1:20
  ☑
  ☑

1) Calculate dB for each Pressure Ratio

- $10^4 / 10^2$
  ☑
- $10^2 / 10^4$
  ☑
- $10^6 / 10^2$
  ☑
- $10^2 / 10^6$
  ☑
- You should now be prepared to solve Practice Problems -- Set 5

2) Given dB, Calculate Pressure Ratio

- 6
  ☑
- 12
  ☑
- 20
  ☑
- 26
  ☑
- 40
  ☑

2) Given dB, Calculate a Pressure Ratio

- 46
  ☑
  ☑

- 52
  ☑
- 0
  ☑

2) Given dB, Calculate a Pressure Ratio

- - 6
  - ☑
  - ☑

- You should now be prepared to solve Practice Problems -- Set 6

3) Given p_x, Calculate dB SPL

- $p_x = 2 \times 10^1$
  - ☑

- $p_x = 4 \times 10^1$
  - ☑
- $p_x = 2 \times 10^2$
  - ☑

3) Given p_x, Calculate dB SPL

- $p_x = 2 \times 10^5$
  - ☑
- $p_x = 10^5$
  - ☑
  - ☑

3) Given p_x, Calculate dB SPL

- $p_x = 2 \times 10^{-2}$
  - ☑

- You should now be prepared to solve Practice Problems -- Set 7

4) Given dB SPL, Calculate p_x

- 0
  - ☑
- 20
  - ☑
  - ☑

4) Given dB SPL, Calculate p_x

- 40
  - ☑
- 46
  - ☑
- 52
  - ☑
- 54
  - ☑

4) Given dB SPL, Calculate p_x

- 80
  - ☑
- 74
  - ☑
  - ☑

- You should now be prepared to solve Practice Problems -- Set 8

Ch4-73

Summary
Four Types of Problems

- 1) Given a pressure ratio, calculate decibels (Set 5)

- 2) Given decibels, calculate pressure ratio (Set 6)

- 3) Given p_x, calculate dB SPL (Set 7)

- 4) Given dB SPL, calculate p_x (Set 8)

Ch4-74

THE RELATION BETWEEN dB IL AND dB SPL

- Intensity ratio of 10:1 = 10 dB, whereas
- Pressure ratio of 10:1 = 20 dB
- Why?
  - ☑
  - ☑

Table 4-2. Relation between decibels for intensity and decibels for pressure

Intensity		Pressure	
Ratio I_x / I_r	dB $10 \log_{10}(I_x / I_r)$	Ratio p_x / p_r	dB $20 \log_{10}(p_x / p_r)$
1	0	1.0000	0
10	**10**	3.1623	10
100	20	**10.0000**	**20**
1,000	30	31.6228	30
10,000	40	100.0000	40
100,000	50	316.2278	50
1,000,000	60	1,000.0000	60

Ch4-75

THE RELATION BETWEEN dB IL AND dB SPL

- Intensity ratio of 2:1 = 3 dB, whereas
- Pressure ratio of 2:1 = 6 dB
- Why?
  - ☑
  - ☑
- 40 dB IL = _dB SPL?
  - ☑

Table 4-2. Relation between decibels for intensity and decibels for pressure

Intensity		Pressure	
Ratio I_x / I_r	dB $10 \log_{10}(I_x / I_r)$	Ratio p_x / p_r	dB $20 \log_{10}(p_x / p_r)$
1	0	1.0000	0
10	**10**	3.1623	10
100	20	**10.0000**	**20**
1,000	30	31.6228	30
10,000	40	100.0000	40
100,000	50	316.2278	50
1,000,000	60	1,000.0000	60

Ch4-76

THE RELATION BETWEEN dB IL AND dB SPL

- If intensity increases by 10:1 (10 dB), pressure increases by the <u>square root of 10:1</u> (3.16:1), and 20 log 3.16 = 10 dB
- Recall:
  - ♦ $p \propto \sqrt{I}$
  - ♦ $I \propto p^2$

Table 4-2. Relation between decibels for intensity and decibels for pressure

Intensity		Pressure	
Ratio I_x / I_r	dB $10 \log_{10}(I_x / I_r)$	Ratio p_x / p_r	dB $20 \log_{10}(p_x / p_r)$
1	0	1.0000	0
10	**10**	3.1623	10
100	20	**10.0000**	**20**
1,000	30	31.6228	30
10,000	40	100.0000	40
100,000	50	316.2278	50
1,000,000	60	1,000.0000	60

Ch4-77

THE RELATION BETWEEN dB IL AND dB SPL

- dB IL = dB SPL because:
- 2×10^1 µPa is the pressure equivalent of 10^{-12} watt / m²
- Thus,
  - ♦ 2×10^1 µPa = 0 dB SPL, and
  - 10^{-12} watt / m² = 0 dB IL

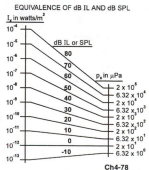

Ch4-78

THE RELATION BETWEEN dB IL AND dB SPL

- 2×10^3 µPa (40 dB SPL) is the pressure equivalent of 10^{-8} watt/m² (40 dB IL)
- More generally, dB IL = dB SPL
- If intensity increases by 2:1,
  - ♦ 3 dB;
- If pressure increases by 2:1,
  - ♦ 6 dB;
- But, if intensity increases by 2:1 (3 dB), pressure increases by only $\sqrt{2:1}$ (3 dB)
- A decibel is a decibel

Ch4-79

UNITS OF MEASURE FOR PRESSURE

- Reference pressures appear in the 0 dB row
- Thus, in 0 dB row,
  - ♦ 2×10^{-4} dyne/cm² (cgs) =
  - ♦ 2×10^{-4} microbar (cgs) =
  - ♦ 2×10^{-5} N/m² (MKS) =
  - ♦ 2×10^{-5} Pa (MKS) =

Table 4-3. Comparisons of various units of measure of pressure

dB SPL	dynes/cm² or microbar	N/m² or Pa	µN/m² or µPa
100	2×10^1	2×10^0	2×10^6
94	10^1	10^0	10^6
80	2×10^0	2×10^{-1}	2×10^5
74	10^0	10^{-1}	10^5
60	2×10^{-1}	2×10^{-2}	2×10^4
54	10^{-1}	10^{-2}	10^4
40	2×10^{-2}	2×10^{-3}	2×10^3
34	10^{-2}	10^{-3}	10^3
20	2×10^{-3}	2×10^{-4}	2×10^2
14	10^{-3}	10^{-4}	10^2
0	2×10^{-4}	2×10^{-5}	2×10^1
-6	10^{-4}	10^{-5}	10^1

UNITS OF MEASURE FOR PRESSURE

- ♦ 2×10^1 µN/m² (MKS) =
- ♦ 2×10^1 µPa (MKS)
- To convert from dyne/cm² (or µbar) to N/m² (or Pa),
  - ♦ divide by 10^1
- To convert from N/m² (or Pa) to µN/m² (or µPa),
  - ♦ multiply by 10^6

Table 4-3. Comparisons of various units of measure of pressure

dB SPL	dynes/cm² or microbar	N/m² or Pa	µN/m² or µPa
100	2×10^1	2×10^0	2×10^6
94	10^1	10^0	10^6
80	2×10^0	2×10^{-1}	2×10^5
74	10^0	10^{-1}	10^5
60	2×10^{-1}	2×10^{-2}	2×10^4
54	10^{-1}	10^{-2}	10^4
40	2×10^{-2}	2×10^{-3}	2×10^3
34	10^{-2}	10^{-3}	10^3
20	2×10^{-3}	2×10^{-4}	2×10^2
14	10^{-3}	10^{-4}	10^2
0	2×10^{-4}	2×10^{-5}	2×10^1
-6	10^{-4}	10^{-5}	10^1

UNITS OF MEASURE OF PRESSURE

- All entries in any given row are equivalent
- For any given column,
  - ♦ A pressure ratio of 2:1 corresponds to 6 dB
  - ♦ A pressure ratio of 10:1 corresponds to 20 dB

Table 4-3. Comparisons of various units of measure of pressure

dB SPL	dynes/cm² or microbar	N/m² or Pa	µN/m² or µPa
100	2×10^1	2×10^0	2×10^6
94	10^1	10^0	10^6
80	2×10^0	2×10^{-1}	2×10^5
74	10^0	10^{-1}	10^5
60	2×10^{-1}	2×10^{-2}	2×10^4
54	10^{-1}	10^{-2}	10^4
40	2×10^{-2}	2×10^{-3}	2×10^3
34	10^{-2}	10^{-3}	10^3
20	2×10^{-3}	2×10^{-4}	2×10^2
14	10^{-3}	10^{-4}	10^2
0	2×10^{-4}	2×10^{-5}	2×10^1
-6	10^{-4}	10^{-5}	10^1

Importantly,

- + dB means that $p_x > p_r$
- 0 dB means that $p_x = p_r$
- - dB means that $p_x < p_r$

Table 4-3. Comparisons of various units of measure of pressure

dB SPL	dynes/cm² or microbar	N/m² or Pa	µN/m² or µPa
100	2×10^1	2×10^0	2×10^6
94	10^1	10^0	10^6
80	2×10^0	2×10^{-1}	2×10^5
74	10^0	10^{-1}	10^5
60	2×10^{-1}	2×10^{-2}	2×10^4
54	10^{-1}	10^{-2}	10^4
40	2×10^{-2}	2×10^{-3}	2×10^3
34	10^{-2}	10^{-3}	10^3
20	2×10^{-3}	2×10^{-4}	2×10^2
14	10^{-3}	10^{-4}	10^2
0	2×10^{-4}	2×10^{-5}	2×10^1
-6	10^{-4}	10^{-5}	10^1

CONVERSION FROM ONE REFERENCE TO ANOTHER

- The equation below enables you to convert between any two reference pressures (p_r) expressed in the same metric system
  - ♦ $dB_{Pr(new)} = dB_{Pr(orig)} - [20 \log_{10}(p_{r(new)} / p_{r(orig)})]$
    where
  - ♦ $p_{r(new)}$ = new reference p_r
    and
  - ♦ $p_{r(orig)}$ = original reference p_r

Ch4-84

CONVERSION FROM ONE REFERENCE TO ANOTHER:
An Example

- For example, 74 dB SPL re: 2×10^{-4} µbar = ? dB re: 1 µbar?
  - ◆ dB SPL = 74 - 20 log $(1 \times 10^{0} / 2 \times 10^{-4})$
  - ◆   = 74 - 20 log $(.5 \times 10^{4})$
  - ◆   = 0

Ch4-85

An Example with Voltage

- 12 dB re: 2v = How many dB re: 1v?
- $dB_{1v} = dB_{2v}$ - [20 $\log_{10}$ (1v / 2v)]
  - ◆ = 12 - (20 log 1 / 2)
  - ◆ = 12 - (- 20 log 2)   {Why?}
  - ☑
  - ◆ = 12 - (- 6)
  - ◆ = 18
  - ◆ Thus, 12 dB re: 2v = 18 dB re: 1v

Ch4-86

COMBINING SOUND INTENSITIES FROM INDEPENDENT SOURCES

- The intensity level of a sound from <u>one</u> noise source is 60 dB IL
- The intensity level of a sound from a <u>second</u>, <u>independent</u> noise source also is 60 dB IL
- If the two noise sources act together, the total intensity level is ?
- ☑

Ch4-87

COMBINING SOUND INTENSITIES FROM INDEPENDENT SOURCES

- If the level from each source is 60 dB IL, then the <u>intensity</u> of each noise must be 10^{-6} watt/m^2 [60 = 10 log ($I_x / 10^{-12}$)]
- If the two sources act together, the <u>total intensity</u> can only be twice as great as the intensity of only one source: 2×10^{-6} watt/m^2

Ch4-88

COMBINING SOUND INTENSITIES FROM INDEPENDENT SOURCES

- Then we see:
  - ◆ dB = 10 log $(2 \times 10^{-6} / 10^{-12})$
  - ◆   = 10 log (2×10^{6})
  - ◆   = 63 dB IL

Ch4-89

COMBINING SOUND INTENSITIES FROM INDEPENDENT SOURCES

- If the intensity level of each source is 60 dB IL, then the <u>sound pressure level</u> of each source must also be 60 dB SPL
- If the intensity level of the two sources combined is 63 dB IL, then the sound pressure level of the two sources combined also is <u>63 dB SPL</u>

Ch4-90

COMBINING SOUND INTENSITIES FROM INDEPENDENT SOURCES

- Why not 66 dB SPL ?
  - ☑

  - ☑

COMBINING SOUND INTENSITIES FROM INDEPENDENT SOURCES

- Two approaches for solving problems in which sound intensities from independent sources are combined
  - ♦ source intensities are equal
  - ♦ source intensities are unequal

A. Equal Source Intensities

- $dB_N = dB_i + 10 \log_{10} N$,
  - ♦ where i = dB SPL (or dB IL) from one source, and
  - ♦ N = # of sources combined

Examples

- 1. Two sources each produce 100 dB SPL. What is the total SPL?
  - ☑

- 2. Three sources each produce 100 dB SPL. What is the total SPL?
  - ☑

Examples

- 3. 1,000 sources each produce 80 dB SPL. What is the total SPL?
  - ☑

- 4. Eight sources each produce 91.2 dB SPL. What is the total SPL?
  - ☑

Examples

- 5. Eight sources each produce 91.2 dB SPL. By how many dB is <u>SPL increased</u>?
  - ☑

B. Unequal Source Intensities

● **Three steps in solution**

   ♦ **1. Calculate intensity from each source**

   ♦ **2. Add intensities (carefully)**

   ♦ **3. Calculate decibels**

Ch4-97

Examples

● **One source = 80 dB SPL, and a second source = 83 dB SPL**

● **<u>dB</u>** $\underline{I}_x$

   ♦ **80** 1×10^{-4}

   ♦ **83** $\underline{2 \times 10^{-4}}$

   ♦ $\Sigma = 3 \times 10^{-4}$

   ♦ **dB = 10 log $(3 \times 10^{-4}) / (10^{-12})$**

      = 10 log (3×10^{8})

      = 84.8 dB IL (dB SPL)
Ch4-98

Examples

● **One source = 80 dB SPL, and a second source = 70 dB SPL**

● **Exponents will be unequal (10^{-4} & 10^{-5}); must express them as equivalent exponents before addition (either - 4 & - 4 or - 5 & - 5)**

●   **<u>dB</u>** $\underline{I}_x$ **<u>Common Exponent</u>**

   ♦ **80** 1×10^{-4} 1×10^{-4}

   ♦ **70** 1×10^{-5} $\underline{0.1 \times 10^{-4}}$

   ♦ $\Sigma = 1.1 \times 10^{-4}$

   ♦ **dB = 10 log $(1.1 \times 10^{-4}) / (10^{-12})$**

      = 80.4 dB IL (dB SPL)
Ch4-99

Summary

● **When combining sound energies from independent sources**

● **It is the energies or powers or intensities that should be added -- not the pressures**

● **Use the "10 - log equation"**

Ch4-100

CHAPTER 5

COMPLEX WAVES

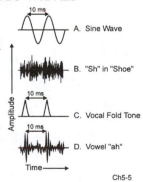

Ch5-1

Preamble

- The sine wave is the fundamental component of all other sound waves
- All waves that are not sinusoidal are <u>complex waves</u>

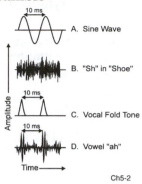

A. Sine Wave

B. "Sh" in "Shoe"

C. Vocal Fold Tone

D. Vowel "ah"

Ch5-2

FOURIER'S THEOREM

- A <u>complex wave</u> is any sound wave that is not sinusoidal
- Complex waves consist of a series of <u>simple sinusoids</u> that can differ in <u>amplitude</u>, <u>frequency</u>, & <u>phase</u>
- This is called a <u>Fourier series</u>
- A Fourier series can be derived by a process that is called <u>Fourier analysis</u>

Ch5-3

Fourier Analysis

- Any complex wave can be decomposed to determine the <u>amplitudes</u>, <u>frequencies</u>, and <u>phases</u> of the sinusoidal components
- <u>All</u> sound waves can be classified by reference to:
  1. Is periodicity present?
  2. How complex is the wave?

Ch5-4

PERIODIC WAVES

- A wave that repeats itself over time
- Also called a <u>periodic time function</u>
- A <u>complex periodic wave</u> is periodic, but not sinusoidal
  - Panels A, C, and D are periodic waves, though panel A is not <u>complex</u> periodic

A. Sine Wave

B. "Sh" in "Shoe"

C. Vocal Fold Tone

D. Vowel "ah"

Ch5-5

Components of a Complex Periodic Wave

- Sinusoidal components cannot be selected at random--They must satisfy an <u>harmonic relation</u>
- With an harmonic relation, each sinusoid in the series must be an <u>integer multiple</u> of the lowest in the series
  - e.g., lowest = 100 Hz: Components are? ☑
  - e.g., lowest = 215 Hz: Components are? ☑

Ch5-6

Harmonic Series

- If harmonic relation is present, the series of components is called an <u>harmonic series</u>

- Each of the components is called an <u>harmonic</u>

  ◆ 1st (and f_0), 2nd, 3rd, 4th, 5th, etc.

Ch5-7

Harmonic Series

- T = 8 ms; f_0 = 125 Hz
- What are the frequencies of the first five harmonics?

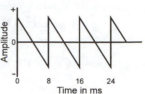

- ☑ 1st (f_0) =
- ☑ 2nd   =
- ☑ 3rd   =
- ☑ 4th   =
- ☑ 5th   =

Ch5-8

Harmonics, Partials, and Overtones

- If all components are <u>exact</u> integer multiples of f_0, harmonic # = partial #
- 2nd harmonic = 1st overtone

Table 5-1. Fundamental frequency, harmonics, partials, and overtones in a complex periodic sound wave

Frequency	Harmonic	Partial	Overtone
125 (f_0)	1	1	
250	2	2	1
375	3	3	2
500	4	4	3
625	5	5	4
750	6	6	5

Ch5-9

Summation of Sine Waves

- Progressive summation of 4 components with identical starting phases
- Each component is an <u>odd</u> integer multiple of f_0
- Compare S_1, C_1, C_2, C_3, & C_∞
- A <u>square wave</u> at ∞

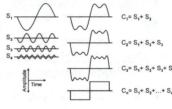

Ch5-10

Summation of Sine Waves

- Progressive summation of 3 components with identical starting phases
- The components are <u>odd & even</u> integer multiples of f_0
- Compare S_1, C_1, C_2, & C_∞
- A <u>sawtooth wave</u> at ∞

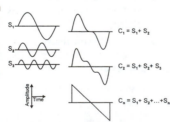

Ch5-11

Summation of Sine Waves

- Summation of two components, S_1 and S_2
  ◆ Starting phase of S_1 is held constant
  ◆ Starting phase of S_2 varies

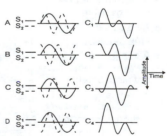

Ch5-12

Summation of Sine Waves

- Note how shape of C changes with changes in starting phase of S_2
  - Panel A: 0°
  - Panel B: 90°
  - Panel C: 180°
  - Panel D: 270°

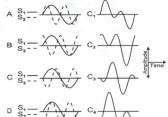

Ch5-13

APERIODIC WAVES

- A wave that lacks periodicity
- Vibratory motion is <u>random</u>, & it sometimes is called a <u>random time function</u>
- Not necessarily "noise"

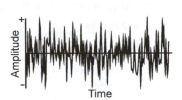

Ch5-14

WAVEFORM AND SPECTRUM

- 1. Waveform
  - Plot of changes in some variable as a function of time
  - e.g., displacement, velocity, acceleration, pressure, etc. as a function of time

Ch5-15

Waveform and Spectrum

- Observe the <u>fundamental period</u>: T = 8 ms
- Can calculate f_0 (125 Hz), but cannot easily see all frequency components, or their amplitudes or starting phases

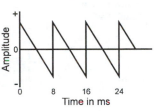

Ch5-16

Waveform and Spectrum

- 2. Amplitude spectrum
  - A graphic alternative to the waveform
  - Also called the amplitude spectrum in the frequency domain

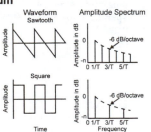

Ch5-17

Waveform and Spectrum

- Shows amplitude as a function of frequency
- The spectral envelope is given by connecting the peaks of the vertical lines: in this case the slope of the envelope is - 6 dB / octave

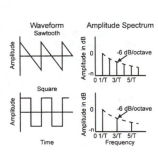

Ch5-18

The Octave

- A doubling of frequency
- A frequency ratio of 2:1 or 1:2
  - ◆ 200:100
  - ◆ 500:250
  - ◆ 4000:2000
  - ◆ 100:200
  - ◆ 250:500
  - ◆ 2000:4000

Ch5-19

Line Spectra

- In these cases, the amplitude spectrum is a <u>line spectrum</u>
  - ◆ Energy <u>only</u> at frequencies identified by vertical lines
  - ◆ Height of vertical line reflects amplitude

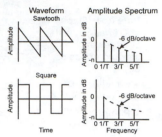

Ch5-20

Continuous Spectra

- Here the amplitude spectrum is a <u>continuous spectrum</u>
  - ◆ Energy present at all frequencies between certain frequency limits
  - ◆ What is slope of envelope?
    ☑
- A slope of 0 dB/octave is not a requirement for continuous spectra

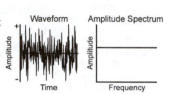

Ch5-21

Waveform and Spectrum

- 3. Phase Spectrum
  - ◆ The phase spectrum in the frequency domain defines the <u>starting phase</u> as a function of frequency
  - ◆ The combination of the amplitude spectrum & the phase spectrum defines the waveform completely in the frequency domain

Ch5-22

EXAMPLES OF COMPLEX WAVES

- Waveforms, amplitude spectra, & phase spectra of four complex waves
- Compare each with the reference sine wave at the top

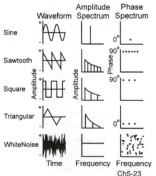

Ch5-23

EXAMPLES OF COMPLEX WAVES

- Can you describe amplitude & phase spectra of the sine wave?
  ☑

  ☑

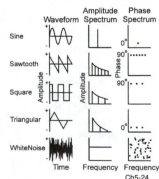

Ch5-24

1. A Sawtooth Wave

- A complex periodic wave with energy at <u>odd</u> and <u>even</u> harmonics that has a <u>spectral envelope slope</u> of - 6 dB / octave
- Amplitudes decrease as the inverse of the harmonic #

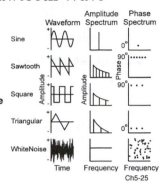

Ch5-25

Sawtooth Wave

- dB = 20 $\log_{10}$ (1 / h_i), where h_i is the harmonic #
- dB = - 20 $\log_{10}$ h_i
- Why?
- ☑

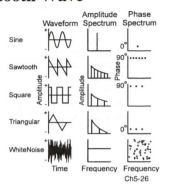

Ch5-26

Sawtooth Wave

- Voltage of f_0 = 2v
- Voltage of other harmonics:
  1/h_i × 2
  - ◆ 2nd harmonic:
    1/2 × 2 = 1 v
  - ◆ 3rd harmonic = ?
  - ☑
  - ◆ 4th harmonic = ?
  - ☑

Table 5-2. Amplitudes (in voltage) of sinusoidal components of a **sawtooth** wave in which the amplitude of the fundamental frequency is 2 V

Harmonic Number	rms voltage (1/ h_i × 2)	-20 $\log_{10}$ h_i
1 (f_0)	1/1 × 2 = 2	0
2	1/2 × 2 = 1	-6
3	1/3 × 2 = .67	-9.5
4	1/4 × 2 = .50	-12
5	1/5 × 2 = .40	-14
6	1/6 × 2 = .33	-15.6
7	1/7 × 2 = .29	-16.9
8	1/8 × 2 = .25	-18.1
9	1/9 × 2 = .22	-19.1

Ch5-27

Sawtooth Wave

- What if voltage of f_0 is 4v?
- What are voltages of 2nd, 3rd, and 4th harmonics?
- ☑
- ☑
- ☑

Table 5-2. Amplitudes (in voltage) of sinusoidal components of a **sawtooth** wave in which the amplitude of the fundamental frequency is 2 V

Harmonic Number	rms voltage (1/ h_i × 2)	-20 $\log_{10}$ h_i
1 (f_0)	1/1 × 2 = 2	0
2	1/2 × 2 = 1	-6
3	1/3 × 2 = .67	-9.5
4	1/4 × 2 = .50	-12
5	1/5 × 2 = .40	-14
6	1/6 × 2 = .33	-15.6
7	1/7 × 2 = .29	-16.9
8	1/8 × 2 = .25	-18.1
9	1/9 × 2 = .22	-19.1

Ch5-28

Sawtooth Wave

- <u>Absolute</u> voltage of any harmonic depends on voltage of f_0!
- <u>Relative level</u>, in dB, is independent of voltage of f_0!
  - ◆ 2nd = - 20 $\log_{10}$ 2 = - 6 dB
  - ◆ 3rd = - 20 $\log_{10}$ 3 = - 9.5 dB
  - ◆ 4th = ?
  - ☑

Ch5-29

Sawtooth Wave

- Comparison among harmonics
  - ◆ 2nd re: 1st (f_0) : - 6 dB
  - ◆ 4th re: 2nd   : - 6 dB
  - ◆ 6th re: 3rd   : - 6 dB
- The spectral envelope slope is - 6 dB / octave

Ch5-30

Sawtooth Wave

- **What does amplitude spectrum of a sawtooth wave "look like?"**
  - ◆ Depends on choice of linear vs. log scales

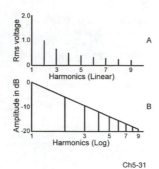

Ch5-31

Summary of Sawtooth Wave

- **A complex periodic wave**
- **Energy at odd & even integer multiples of f_0**
- **Spectral envelope slope of - 6 dB/octave**
- **dB = $20 \log_{10} (1/h_i)$ = - $20 \log_{10} h_i$**

Ch5-32

2. Square Wave

- **A complex periodic wave with energy only at <u>odd</u> integer multiples of f_0 that has a spectral envelope slope of - 6 dB/octave**

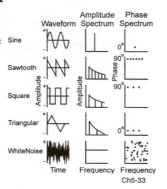

Ch5-33

Square Wave

- **Amplitudes decrease as the inverse of the harmonic #**
- **dB = $20 \log_{10} (1/h_i)$ = - $20 \log_{10} h_i$**

Table 5-3. Amplitudes (in voltage) of sinusoidal components of a **square** wave in which the amplitude of the fundamental frequency is 2 V

Harmonic Number	rms voltage $(1/h_i \times 2)$	- $20 \log_{10} h_i$
1 (f_0)	$1/1 \times 2 = 2$	0
3	$1/3 \times 2 = .67$	-9.5
5	$1/5 \times 2 = .40$	-14
7	$1/7 \times 2 = .29$	-16.9
9	$1/9 \times 2 = .22$	-19.1

Ch5-34

Summary of Square Wave

- **Complex periodic wave**
- **Energy only at <u>odd</u> integer multiples of f_0**
- **Spectral envelope slope of - 6 dB/octave**
- **dB = $20 \log_{10} (1/h_i)$ = - $20 \log_{10} h_i$**

Ch5-35

Summary of Square Wave

- **What about the phase spectrum?**
- **Confusion among textbooks**
  - ◆ **Some will show the starting phase to be 0°; others as 90°**
  - ◆ **Each is correct, but all harmonics must have the same starting phase**

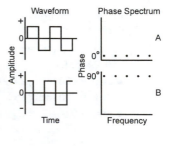

Ch5-36

3. Triangular Wave

- A complex periodic wave with energy only at <u>odd</u> harmonics
- What distinguishes the triangular wave from the square wave?

☑

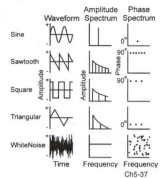

Ch5-37

Triangular Wave

- Amplitudes decrease as the <u>reciprocal of the square</u> of the harmonic #
- dB = $20 \log_{10} 1/h_i^2$
  = $-20 \log_{10} h_i^2$
  = $-40 \log_{10} h_i$
- Why -40?

☑

Table 5-4. Amplitudes (in voltage) of sinusoidal components of a **triangular** wave in which the amplitude of the fundamental frequency is 2 V

Harmonic Number	rms voltage $(1/h_i^2 \times 2)$	$-40 \log_{10} h_i$
1 (f_0)	$1/1^2 \times 2 = 2$	0
3	$1/3^2 \times 2 = .22$	-19.1
5	$1/5^2 \times 2 = .08$	-28
7	$1/7^2 \times 2 = .04$	-33.8
9	$1/9^2 \times 2 = .025$	-38.2

Ch5-38

Triangular Wave

- We saw earlier that the 5th harmonic of a square or sawtooth wave was -14 dB
- But, the 5th harmonic of triangular wave is -28 dB ($20 \log_{10} 1/5^2$)
- The spectral envelope slope is -12 dB / octave

Table 5-4. Amplitudes (in voltage) of sinusoidal components of a **triangular** wave in which the amplitude of the fundamental frequency is 2 V

Harmonic Number	rms voltage $(1/h_i^2 \times 2)$	$-40 \log_{10} h_i$
1 (f_0)	$1/1^2 \times 2 = 2$	0
3	$1/3^2 \times 2 = .22$	-19.1
5	$1/5^2 \times 2 = .08$	-28
7	$1/7^2 \times 2 = .04$	-33.8
9	$1/9^2 \times 2 = .025$	-38.2

Ch5-39

Summary of Triangular Wave

- Complex periodic wave
- Energy only at <u>odd</u> integer multiples of f_0
- Spectral envelope slope of -12 dB / octave
- dB = $20 \log_{10} (1/h_i^2) = -40 \log_{10} h_i$

Ch5-40

4. Pulse Train

- A repetitious series of rectangularly shaped pulses
- Each pulse has some width or duration (P_d)
- Is it periodic or aperiodic?

☑

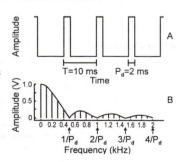

Ch5-41

Pulse Train

- In this example, P_d = 2 ms
- The period (T) of the pulse is 10 ms
- 1/T defines the <u>pulse repetition frequency</u> (PRF): PRF = ?

☑

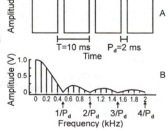

Ch5-42

Pulse Train

- A complex periodic wave with <u>harmonics</u> at odd and even integer multiples of the pulse repetition frequency: 100, 200, 300, etc.
- Amplitude spectrum shows <u>lobes</u> and <u>valleys (nulls)</u>
- <u>Nulls</u> occur at integer multiples of reciprocal of P_d

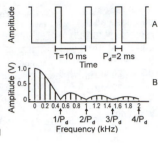

Ch5-43

Pulse Train

- Thus, nulls occur at $1/P_d$, $2/P_d$, $3/P_d$, etc.
  - ◆ 500 Hz, 1000 Hz, 1500 Hz
- Starting phases?
  - ◆ Below 1st null: 0°
  - ◆ Between 1st and 2nd null: 180°
  - ◆ Between 2nd and 3rd null: 0°
  - ◆ and so forth

Ch5-44

5. White, or Gaussian, Noise

- An aperiodic waveform with equal energy in every frequency band 1 Hz wide: from
  - ◆ f - 0.5 Hz to f + 0.5 Hz
- Why is this noise called "white noise"?
  - ◆ Analogous to white light -- equal energy in all light wavelengths

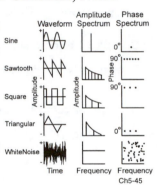

Ch5-45

Why is White Noise Called Gaussian Noise?

- A random time function can be described by a <u>cumulative probability distribution</u> (left)
- A plot of the changing slope of a cumulative probability distribution is called a <u>probability density function</u> (right)

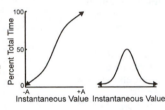

Ch5-46

Why is White Noise Called Gaussian Noise?

- For white noise, the probability density function is a <u>normal curve</u>, or Gaussian distribution
- Spectral envelope slope of 0 dB/octave
- Starting phases in random array

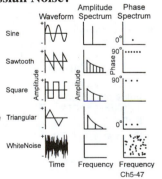

Ch5-47

6. A Single Pulse

- $P_d = 2$ ms
- Is the waveform periodic?
  - ☑
  - ☑

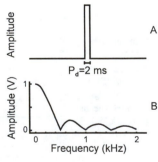

Ch5-48

Pulse Train (Revisited)

● T (ms)	● PRF (Hz)
◆ 10	◆ 100
◆ 20	◆ 50
◆ 40	◆ 25
◆ 80	◆ 12.5
◆ 160	◆ 6.25
◆ 320	◆ 3.125
◆ ∞	◆ 0

- At T = ∞, PRF = 0 and the spacing between harmonics = 0
- The result is a continuous spectrum
- Nulls still occur at $1/P_d$, $2/P_d$, $3/P_d$, etc.

Ch5-49

MEASURES OF SOUND PRESSURE FOR COMPLEX WAVES

- Different equations required for different signals
- True rms meter vs. average-responding meter
- Only the true rms meter will correctly read the rms voltage of signals other than sinusoids

Table 5-5. Measures of sound pressure for sine, square, and random waveforms. **A** refers to the peak or **maximum amplitude** as defined in Chapter 2

Metrics	Types of Waveforms		
	Sine	Square	Random
rms	$\dfrac{A}{\sqrt{2}}$	A	~ 0.3 A
mean square	$\dfrac{A^2}{2}$	A^2	~ 0.1 A
FW$_{avg}$	$\dfrac{2A}{\pi}$	A	~ .25 A
peak	A	A	A

Ch5-50

SIGNAL-TO-NOISE RATIO IN dB (dB S/N)

- It is the ratio of signal level to noise level
- dB S / N = $10 \log_{10} (I_S/I_N)$
- If S = 70 dB and N = 66 dB
  - ◆ dB S / N = 4 dB
- Why?
  - ☑

  - ☑

  - ☑

Ch5-51

CHAPTER 6

RESONANCE AND FILTERING

Ch6-1

Preamble

- Signal is complex-periodic with a fundamental frequency and harmonics
- Volume velocity refers to the particle velocity of air molecules flowing through an area of $1 \, m^3/s$
  - A line spectrum
  - **Smooth** envelope with no sharp prominences

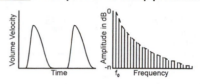

Ch6-2

Preamble

- Sounds similar to a "buzz"
- Produced by vibration of vocal folds during, e.g., vowel production
- The sound wave will be altered or "reinforced" by a process called <u>resonance</u>, or <u>filtering</u>, to produce the various vowels of the language

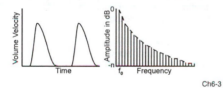

Ch6-3

Preamble

- Thus, through the process of resonance, the vocal fold source spectrum is modified, selectively, to become
  - /i/ as in b<u>ea</u>t
  - /u/ as in b<u>oo</u>t
  - and so forth

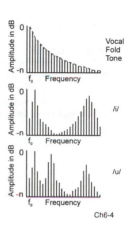

Ch6-4

RESONANCE

- What is resonance, and why does it occur?
- Strike a tuning fork; it vibrates at its own natural frequency, f_{nat}, which is governed by the mass and stiffness of the fork
- Touch the vibrating fork to some hard surface
  - Pitch is unaltered but loudness increases: Why?
  - Explained by the "Principle of Resonance"

Ch6-5

The Principle of Resonance

- Periodic force (vibrating fork) is applied to an elastic system (hard surface)
- System is <u>forced</u> to vibrate at frequency of applied force, not at f_{nat} of the system
- The closer the frequency of the <u>applied force</u> to the <u>natural frequency</u> (f_{nat}) of the system, the <u>greater</u> the <u>amplitude</u> of vibration (loudness increases)

Ch6-6

A Comparison of Two Elastic Systems

- Sinusoids with variable frequency, <u>but with constant amplitude</u>, are directed to two different elastic systems (A & B)
- At output of systems, amplitudes <u>vary</u> with frequency

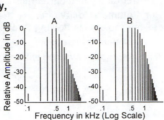

Ch6-7

A Comparison of Two Elastic Systems

- Greatest amplitude occurs at f_{nat} of the elastic system
- What does 0 dB mean?
  ☑

- In A, what is the natural frequency?
  ☑

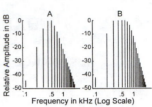

Ch6-8

A Comparison of Two Elastic Systems

- What happens at frequencies remote from the natural frequency?
  ☑
- How are the two displays similar and different?
  ☑

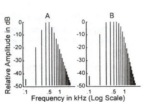

Ch6-9

RESONANCE AND FILTER CURVES

- The figure does not represent a sound wave
- The curve describes a frequency-selective elastic system
- It shows the relative amplitude of forced vibrations as a function of frequency that would be realized if driving forces of variable frequency, but constant amplitude, were applied

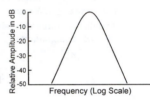

Ch6-10

RESONANCE AND FILTER CURVES

- The curve is called:
  - ♦ Resonance curve
  - ♦ Filter curve
  - ♦ System transfer function
  - ♦ Amplitude response
  - ♦ "Frequency response"

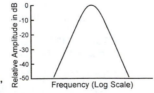

Ch6-11

RESONANCE AND FILTER CURVES

- Note the <u>natural frequency</u> at 0 dB
- What happens above & below the natural frequency?
  ☑

- The resonator, or filter, is a <u>frequency-selective system</u>

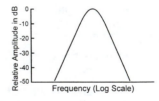

Ch6-12

Summary

- Mass and stiffness of elastic system determine its <u>natural</u>, or <u>resonant</u>, <u>frequency</u>
- Elastic system is forced to vibrate at frequency of applied force
- Amplitude of vibration of elastic system is greatest when <u>driving frequency</u> equals <u>natural frequency</u> of system
- Why? Review impedance

Ch6-13

ACOUSTIC IMPEDANCE & RESONANCE

- Two components of impedance (Z):
  - ◆ Energy dissipating - Resistance (R)
  - ◆ Energy storage   - Reactance (X)
- The magnitude of resistance (R) is independent of frequency
  - ◆ Thus, R does not contribute to determination of f_{nat}
- What components of Z, therefore, determine f_{nat}?
  - ☑
  - ☑

Ch6-14

Reactance (X)

- Reactance is <u>frequency dependent</u>
  - ◆ Mass reactance (X_m) is <u>directly</u> proportional to frequency
    >>$X_m \propto f$
    >>$X_m = 2\pi fm$

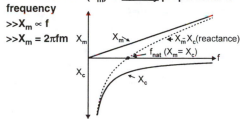

Ch6-15

Reactance (X)

- ◆ Compliant reactance (X_c) is <u>inversely</u> proportional to frequency
  >>$X_c \propto 1/f$
  >>$X_c = 1/2\pi fc$

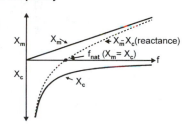

Ch6-16

Reactance (X)

- What if $X_m = X_c$?
  - ◆ X = 0
  - ◆ Z = R
  - ◆ Z is minimal
  - ◆ Amplitude of vibration is greatest
- The frequency at which $X_m = X_c$, where Z is minimal (Z = R) and amplitude is greatest, is the natural frequency, f_{nat}

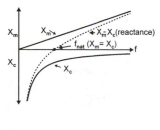

Ch6-17

Mass Reactance (X_m) and Compliant Reactance (X_c)

- If $f < f_{nat}$?
  - ◆Z increases
  - ◆Amplitude of vibration decreases
  - ◆Compliance dominant ($X_c = 1/2\pi fc$)

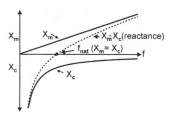

Ch6-18

Mass Reactance (X_m) and Compliant Reactance (X_c)

- If $f > f_{nat}$?
  - ◆ Z increases
  - ◆ Amplitude of vibration decreases
  - ◆ Mass dominant ($X_m = 2\pi f m$)

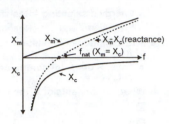

Ch6-19

Effects of Impedance on Resonance Curve

- Shape of resonance curve, & location in frequency domain, determined by <u>impedance</u> (Z) of resonant system: The relative contributions of R, X_m, & X_c

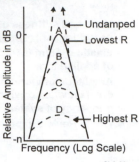

Ch6-20

Effects of Impedance on Resonance Curve

- Dashed curve (labeled "undamped"): No R
  - ◆ Infinite response of system at f_{nat}
  - ◆ $X_m = X_c$; R = 0
- Curve A
  - ◆ R limits maximum amplitude
  - ◆ Peak amplitude occurs at f_{nat} where $X_m = X_c$

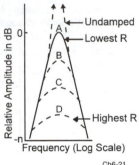

Ch6-21

Effects of Impedance on Resonance Curve

- ◆ At <u>natural frequency</u> (f_{nat} or f_c), $X_m = X_c$, and Z is determined only by R
- ◆ At <u>natural frequency</u>, system is "set into resonance"

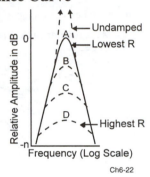

Ch6-22

Effects of Impedance on Resonance Curve

- ◆ Below f_c : <u>compliance dominant</u> (Why?)
  - ☑
- ◆ Above f_c : <u>mass dominant</u> (Why?)
  - ☑

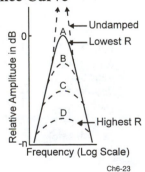

Ch6-23

Effects of Impedance on Resonance Curve

- ● Curves B, C, & D
  - ◆ Progressive increase of <u>resistance</u>, not just impedance
  - ◆ Is natural frequency affected?
    - ☑

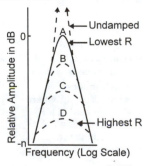

Ch6-24

Effects of Impedance on Resonance Curve

- As R increases from B to C to D:
  - ◆ More energy is dissipated
  - ◆ Damping increases
  - ◆ System becomes more <u>broadly</u> <u>tuned</u>

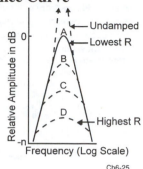

Ch6-25

Admittance

- <u>Impedance</u> emphasizes opposition to motion; opposition to transfer of energy

- <u>Admittance</u> refers to the inverse; energy accepted, or admitted, to a system

Ch6-26

Admittance

- Admittance is inversely proportional to Z, hence Z^{-1}
- Units of Measure
  - ◆ Ohm Z   (impedance)
  - ◆ Mho Z^{-1} (admittance)
  - ◆ Why Z^{-1}?
    - ☑
    - ☑

Ch6-27

System Tuning

- The figure compares two resonant systems (not signals)
- Narrow tuning at left
- <u>Good generator</u> of sound: Why?
  - ◆ lower resistance
  - ◆ less damping
  - ◆ longer free vibrations at f_{nat}

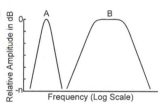

Ch6-28

System Tuning

- Broad tuning at right
- <u>Good receiver</u> of sound: Why?
  - ◆ higher resistance
  - ◆ more damping
  - ◆ brief free vibrations
  - ◆ can be forced to vibrate with maximum amplitude over a wide range of frequencies

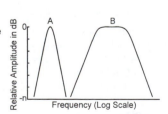

Ch6-29

Impedance Matching

- Apply vibrating force (driver) to elastic system (load)
  - ◆ Power transferred to system
  - ◆ System forced to vibrate
- <u>Maximum amplitude</u> occurs at f_c where Z is minimal and Z^{-1} is maximal
- Maximum power transfer occurs when Z of driver = Z of load

Ch6-30

Examples of Impedance Matching

- Sounding board of a piano
- Air cavity above the vocal folds
  - ◆ Do <u>not</u> amplify sound
  - ◆ Zs are matched
  - ◆ <u>Maximum</u> transfer of power

Ch6-31

FREQUENCY-SELECTIVE SYSTEMS: FILTERS

- A: Amplitude spectrum of input signal
- B: System transfer function (resonance, or filter, curve)
  - ◆ Peak occurs at f_c (f_{nat}) where $X_m = X_c$
  - ◆ Curve shows how amplitudes of input signal <u>will be</u> attenuated as a function of frequency

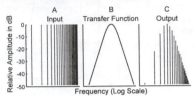

Ch6-32

FREQUENCY-SELECTIVE SYSTEMS: FILTERS

- C: Amplitude spectrum of output signal
  - ◆ Harmonic with $f = f_c$ has greatest amplitude: Why?
    - ☑

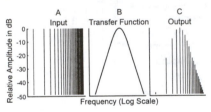

Ch6-33

FREQUENCY-SELECTIVE SYSTEMS: FILTERS

- ◆ Harmonics > f_c are progressively attenuated: Why?
  - ☑
  - ☑
- ◆ Harmonics < f_c are progressively attenuated: Why?
  - ☑
  - ☑

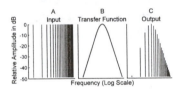

Ch6-34

FREQUENCY-SELECTIVE SYSTEMS: FILTERS

- A: Amplitude spectrum of input signal -- white noise
- B: Transfer function of system
- C: Amplitude spectrum of output signal
  - ◆ Frequency-limited (band-limited) white noise

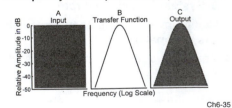

Ch6-35

PARAMETERS OF A FILTER (SYSTEM TRANSFER FUNCTION)

- Two filter curves
- Five principal parameters of filter curves
  - ◆ 1. Center (natural) frequency, f_c
  - ◆ 2. Upper cutoff frequency, f_U

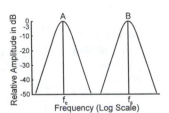

Ch6-36

PARAMETERS OF A FILTER (SYSTEM TRANSFER FUNCTION)

- ◆ 3. Lower cutoff frequency, f_L
- ◆ 4. Bandwidth, Δf
- ◆ 5. Attenuation (rejection) rate

Ch6-37

1. Center (Natural) Frequency (f_c)

- Frequency corresponding to maximum amplitude of vibration, f_c
  - ◆ At f_c, $X_m = X_c$
- Compare two curves
  - ◆ Z is minimal at f_c
  - ◆ Z^{-1} is maximal at f_c
- Contrast two curves
  - ◆ $f_c(B) > f_c(A)$

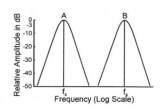

Ch6-38

2. Upper Cutoff Frequency (f_U)

- That frequency <u>above</u> f_c for which amplitude of response is 3 dB less than response at f_c
- The 3-dB down point or the half-power point
- Why is it called the 3-dB down point?
  - ☑

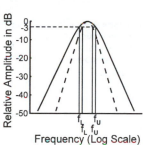

Ch6-39

3. Lower Cutoff Frequency (f_L)

- How would you define f_L?
  - ☑

- The 3-dB down point or the half-power point: Why?
  - ☑

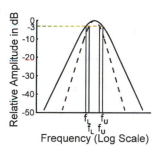

Ch6-40

4. Bandwidth (Δf or BW)

- Δf defines the <u>passband</u> of the system: the range of frequencies <u>passed</u> by the filter
- $\Delta f = f_U - f_L$
- Δf quantifies how narrowly or broadly tuned the filter is

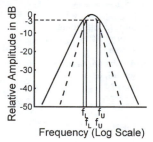

Ch6-41

5. Attenuation Rate In dB/octave

- Attenuation rate
  - ◆ Roll-off rate
  - ◆ Rejection rate
- The rate at which energy for frequencies < f_c or > f_c is rejected (attenuated)
- The slope of the filter curve, expressed in dB/octave

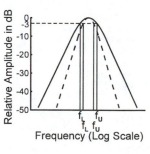

Ch6-42

Attenuation Rate In dB/octave

- Filter A:
  10 dB/octave
- Filter B:
  15 dB/octave
- Attenuation rate quantifies the "selectivity" of a filter

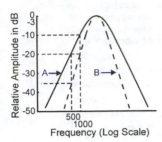

Ch6-43

IDEALIZED VS. REALIZED FILTER

- When we specify parameters of a real filter, we describe it as if it were an idealized rectangular filter (blue)
- Specification of attenuation rate reveals how much the realized filter (black) departs from the idealized one

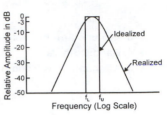

Ch6-44

FOUR TYPES OF FILTERS

1. **Low-Pass**

2. **High-Pass**

3. **Band-Pass**

4. **Band-Reject**

Ch6-45

1. Low-Pass Filter

- <u>Passes</u> energy <u>below</u> some f_U: attenuates energy above f_U
- Two parameters:
  - f_U
  - Attenuation rate
- What is Δf ?
  ☑

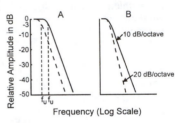

Ch6-46

2. High-Pass Filter

- <u>Passes</u> energy <u>above</u> some f_L: attenuates energy below f_L
- Two parameters; what are they?
  ☑
  ☑
- What is Δf ?
  - $\Delta f = \Delta f_{sig} - f_L$

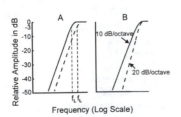

Ch6-47

3. Band-Pass Filter

- <u>Passes</u> energy <u>between</u> some f_L and f_U: attenuates energy below f_L and above f_U
- All five parameters useful; what are they?
  ☑
- What is Δf?
  ☑

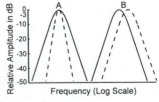

Ch6-48

Band-Pass Filter

- A band-pass filter is a combination of a low-pass & high-pass filter connected <u>in series</u>

-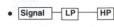

  ♦ or vice versa

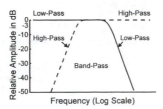

Ch6-49

TWO TYPES OF BAND-PASS FILTERS

a. Band - Pass

b. Constant Percentage Bandwidth

Ch6-50

a. Band-Pass Filter

- Δf is independent of f_c
- Panel A: Amplitude spectrum of input signal, white noise, X
- Panel B: Two transfer functions, Y & Z
  ♦ $\Delta f_Y = \Delta f_Z$
- Why do bandwidths of Y and Z appear to be different?
  ☑

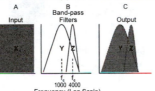

Ch6-51

Band-Pass Filter

- Panel C: Amplitude spectrum of two band-limited output signals, Y & Z
- Levels in dB
  ♦ X_{dB} = input level
  ♦ Y_{dB} = output level from filter Y
  ♦ Z_{dB} = output level from filter Z

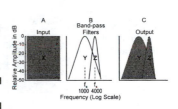

Ch6-52

Band-Pass Filter

- $Y_{dB} < X_{dB}$ Why?
  ☑

- $Z_{dB} < X_{dB}$ Why?
  ☑

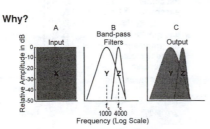

Ch6-53

Band-Pass Filter

- $Y_{dB} = Z_{dB}$ Why?
  ☑
  ☑

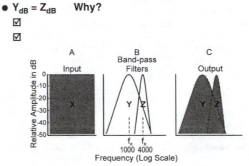

Ch6-54

b. Constant Percentage Bandwidth Filter

- The bandwidth, Δf, is <u>always</u> a constant percentage of the center frequency, f_c; Δf is <u>not</u> independent of f_c

- Consider sales tax analogy

  - Let purchase price be analogous to f_c and tax be analogous to Δf

  - As purchase price increases by some factor, say 10:1, tax owed increases by same factor, 10:1

Ch6-55

Constant Percentage Bandwidth Filter

- Suppose constant % is 70.7
- Thus, $\Delta f = .707(f_c)$
- Calculations
  - Δf for Y = ?
    >> 0.707 (1000)
    = 707 Hz
  - Δf for Z = ?
    >> 0.707 (4000)
    = 2828 Hz

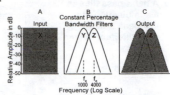

Ch6-56

Constant Percentage Bandwidth Filter

- Why do the two filters <u>appear</u> to have the same bandwidth?
  ☑

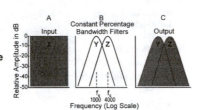

Ch6-57

Constant Percentage Bandwidth Filter

- As before,
  - $Y_{dB} < X_{dB}$ Why?
    ☑

  - $Z_{dB} < X_{dB}$ Why?
    ☑

- Important point!
  - $Z_{dB} > Y_{dB}$ Why?
    ☑

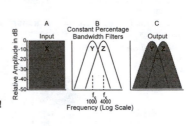

Ch6-58

Common Constant Percentage Bandwidth Filters

- One-octave (1/1) filter
  - $\Delta f = .707 \times f_c$
  - $f_L = .707 \times f_c$
  - $f_U = 1.414 \times f_c$ Why?
    ☑

- As f_c changes by some factor, f_L, f_U, and Δf change by the same factor!

Table 6-1. Lower cutoff frequency (f_L), upper cutoff frequency (f_U), and bandwidth (Δf) for various values of the center frequency (f_c) for a one-octave filter

f_c	f_L	f_U	$\Delta f = f_U - f_L$
100	70.7	141.4	70.7
200	141.4	282.8	141.4
1000	707	1414	707
2000	1414	2828	1414
10,000	7070	14,140	7070

Ch6-59

Common Constant Percentage Bandwidth Filters

- A one-octave filter
- f_c appears to be at the center of passband, and <u>it is on a log scale</u>
- It is <u>not</u>, however, the arithmetic mean of the two cutoff frequencies
- It is the <u>geometric mean</u>
  - $G = \sqrt[N]{x_1 \cdot x_2 \cdot \ldots \cdot x_N}$
  - $f_c = \sqrt{f_L \cdot f_U}$

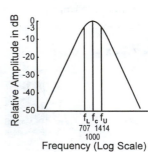

Ch6-60

Common Constant Percentage Bandwidth Filters

- 1/1, 1/2, 1/3, 1/10
- A 1/n filter, where
  - n is the denominator in the fraction
- Note how bandwidth (Δf) changes with changes in 1/n

Table 6-2. Parameters of various constant percentage bandwidth filters. The center frequency is a constant 1000 Hz

1/n	f_c	f_L	f_U	Δf	%
1/1	1000	707	1414	707	70.7
1/2	1000	844	1190	346	34.6
1/3	1000	891	1122	231	23.1
1/10	1000	966	1035	69	6.9

- $f_L = \text{antilog}_{10}(\log_{10}[f_c - .3/2n])$,
- $f_U = \text{antilog}_{10}(\log_{10}[f_c + .3/2n])$
- $\Delta f = f_U - f_L$

Ch6-61

Preferred Center Frequencies for 1/10-, 1/3-, and 1/1-Octave Filters

- All values of f_c in Table 6-3 apply to 1/10 & 1/3 filters; bold face values in parentheses are preferred for a 1/1 filter
- The preferred values differ by a constant ratio

  >> For 1/10 and 1/3, the base is 1.25

  >> For 1/1, the base is 2

Ch6-62

- ANSI S1.6-1984, revised 1997. Copyright by Acoustical Society of America. **Not for resale**. No part of this publication may be copied or reproduced in any form, including electronic retrieval system or be made available on the Internet, a public network, by satellite or otherwise without the prior written permission of the Acoustical Society of America, 120 Wall Street, 32nd Floor, NY,NY 10005-3993 USA. Phone (212) 248-0373, Fax (212) 248-0146, E-mail: asastds@aip.org

Table 6-3. Frequency band numbers (**N**) and preferred center frequencies (f_c) for nominal 1/3- or 1/10-octave filters and for 1-octave filters (boldface only).* Values below band 20 and above band 40 have not been included

N	f_c	N	f_c
20	100		
21	(125)	31	1250
22	160	32	1600
23	200	33	(2000)
24	(250)	34	2500
25	315	35	3150
26	400	36	(4000)
27	(500)	37	5000
28	630	38	6300
29	800	39	(8000)
30	(1000)	40	10,000

Ch6-63

4. Band-Reject Filter

- <u>Rejects</u> energy <u>between</u> some f_L and f_U
- A band-reject filter is a combination of a low-pass & high-pass filter connected <u>in parallel</u>

-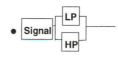

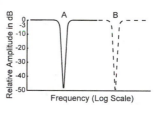

Ch6-64

SPECIFICATION OF LEVEL AT THE OUTPUT OF FILTERS

- Level at output of filter is reduced because <u>energy is attenuated selectively as a function of frequency</u>
- We will use a white noise signal, which has equal energy per cycle, as the input signal for computational convenience in all calculations
- To proceed, we need to introduce the concept of <u>pressure spectrum level</u>, **L**$_{ps}$

Ch6-65

Pressure Spectrum Level, L_{ps}

- L_{ps} is the sound pressure level in <u>any</u> frequency band 1 Hz wide
- Relate to white noise: White noise has a pressure spectrum level slope of 0 dB

Ch6-66

Pressure Spectrum Level, L_{ps}

- Equation 6.9

  $L_{ps} = SPL_{wb} - 10 \log_{10} (\Delta f_{wb}/\Delta_o f)$

- Equation 6.10 (6.9 simplified)

  $L_{ps} = SPL_{wb} - 10 \log_{10} \Delta f_{wb}$

- How is simplification in 6.10 justified?

  ☑

Ch6-67

Pressure Spectrum Level, L_{ps} (Sample Problem)

- A white noise signal with $\Delta f = 10,000$ Hz has SPL = 75 dB

- Think of white noise being filtered with an <u>idealized rectangular filter</u> with $\Delta f = 1$ Hz

- What is L_{ps}?

  ☑

Ch6-68

Pressure Spectrum Level, L_{ps}

☑

☑

☑

☑

- What is p_r for L_{ps} ?

  ☑

Ch6-69

Pressure Spectrum Level, L_{ps}

- Suppose we are given L_{ps} and Δf of signal

- Could we calculate overall SPL?

  ☑

  ☑

Ch6-70

Pressure Spectrum Level, L_{ps} (Sample Problem)

- A white noise signal has a bandwidth of 10,000 Hz and a pressure spectrum level, L_{ps}, of 42 dB SPL

- What is the overall level?

  ☑

Ch6-71

Pressure Spectrum Level, L_{ps}

- Relate L_{ps} to concept of white noise
  - ◆ By definition: The level in any frequency band 1 Hz wide is the same -- regardless of the value of f
  - ◆ Think of each band 1 Hz wide as an independent source of sound
  - ◆ Then apply equation 4.9

    >> $dB_N = dB_i + 10 \log_{10} N$

    >> $dB_{wb} = L_{ps} + 10 \log_{10} \Delta f_{wb}$ (parallel concept)

Ch6-72

Sample Problems

- White noise signal has Δf = 5000 Hz and overall SPL = 75 dB

- What is L_{ps}?

  ☑

Ch6-73

Sample Problems

- White noise signal has Δf = 8000 Hz and pressure spectrum level of 40 dB SPL

- What is overall level?

  ☑

Ch6-74

The More General Case

- A representation of Δf
  - At bottom, Δf = 1 Hz
  - Δf increases to 10,000 Hz & beyond
- Can calculate <u>any</u> SPL_{nb} from <u>any</u> SPL_{wb}, and vice versa

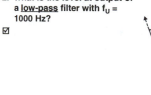

Ch6-75

The More General Case

- Equation 6.12 (a variation of Equation 6.10)
  - $SPL_{nb} = SPL_{wb} - 10 \log_{10} (\Delta f_{wb} / \Delta f_{nb})$
- Equation 6.13 (a variation of Equation 6.11)
  - $SPL_{wb} = SPL_{nb} + 10 \log_{10} (\Delta f_{wb} / \Delta f_{nb})$

Ch6-76

Sample Problems

- A white noise has a bandwidth of 10,000 Hz and an overall level of 90 dB SPL
- 1. What is the level at the output of <u>band-pass</u> filter with Δf = 1000 Hz?

  ☑

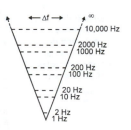

Ch6-77

Sample Problems

- 2. What is the level at output of a <u>low-pass</u> filter with f_U = 1000 Hz?

  ☑

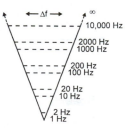

  ☑

Ch6-78

Sample Problems

● 3. What is the level at output of a
   <u>low-pass</u> filter with f_U = 2000 Hz?

☑

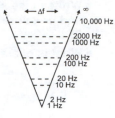

Ch6-79

Sample Problems

● 4. What is level at output of a <u>one-octave</u>
   filter with f_c = 1414 Hz?

☑

Ch6-80

Sample Problems

● 5. What is level at output of a <u>one-octave</u>
   filter with f_c = 2828 Hz?

● What is the most simple approach?

☑

● What other avenues are available?

☑

☑

Ch6-81

Sample Problems

● 6. What is level at output of a <u>high-pass</u>
   filter with f_L = 9000 Hz?

☑

Ch6-82

SELECTED NOISES AND SPEECH

● White Noise

● Pink Noise

● Speech

Ch6-83

White Noise

● By definition, the
level in any
frequency band 1
Hz wide is the
same regardless
of the value of f

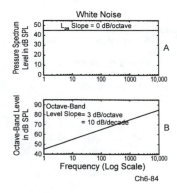

Ch6-84

White Noise

- Panel A: Ordinate is L_{ps} (L_{ps} = 45 dB SPL)
- White noise has a pressure spectrum level slope of 0 dB
- Panel B: Filter the white noise with a 1/1-octave filter at several values of f_c

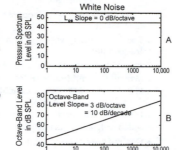

Ch6-85

White Noise

- Call the readings <u>octave-band levels</u>
- At 100 Hz, octave-band level is 63.5 dB SPL
  - ♦ $\Delta f_{70.7}$ = 45 + 10 log 70.7 = 63.5   (6.11)
- What will you read at 200, 400, 800 Hz, etc.?
  - ☑
  - ☑
  - ☑

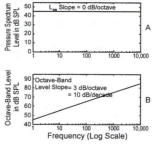

Ch6-86

White Noise

- What will you read at 10 Hz & 1000 Hz?
  - ☑

  - ☑

White Noise

Ch6-87

White Noise

- Plot the results as shown in Panel B where the ordinate now is octave-band level in dB SPL
- White noise has an <u>octave-band level slope</u> of:
  - ♦ +3 dB / octave, or
  - ♦ +10 dB / decade
- White noise has a <u>pressure spectrum level slope</u> of 0 dB (Panel A)

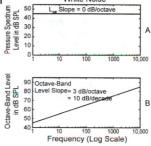

Ch6-88

Pink Noise

- By definition, pink noise has an <u>octave-band level slope</u> of 0 dB (Panel B)
- Pink noise has a <u>pressure spectrum level slope</u> of:
  - ♦ - 3 dB / octave
  - ♦ -10 dB / decade (Panel A)

Pink Noise

Ch6-89

Calculations of Pressure Spectrum Levels for Pink Noise

- For all values of f_c, the octave-band levels in the example are 45 dB SPL
- Calculate L_{ps} for two values of f_c with a frequency ratio of 2:1
  - ♦ f_c = 100 Hz: Δf = ? L_{ps} = ?
    - ☑
    - ☑

  - ♦ f_c = 200 Hz : Δf = ? L_{ps} = ?
    - ☑
    - ☑

- Slope = - 3 dB / octave

Ch6-90

Calculations of Pressure Spectrum Levels for Pink Noise

- Calculate L_{ps} for two values of f_c with a frequency ratio of 10:1
    - f_c = 100 Hz : Δf = ? L_{ps} = ?
        - ☑
        - ☑
    - f_c = 1000 Hz : Δf = ? L_{ps} = ?
        - ☑
        - ☑
- Slope = -10 dB / octave

Ch6-91

Amplitude Spectrum of Connected Speech

- Passage of Connected Discourse Spoken by One Talker (Male)
    - Speech intensity varies over time and across frequencies
- Measurement procedure
    - Measure output (voltage) from 1/3-octave filters with f_c set to <u>preferred frequencies</u> from f_c = 100 Hz (Δf = 23.1 Hz) to f_c = 10,000 Hz (Δf = 2310 Hz)
    - Make several hundred measurements for each value of f_c and average
    - Results are called <u>one-third octave-band levels</u>
    - From each one-third octave-band level, compute L_{ps} (6.10)

Ch6-92

Amplitude Spectrum of Connected Speech

- Result
    - open circles: one-third octave-band levels
    - blue circles: L_{ps}
- Note how curves diverge with increasing f_c: Why?
    - ☑

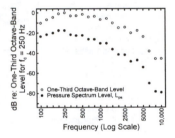

Ch6-93

Amplitude Spectrum of Connected Speech

- For f_c = 100 Hz (Δf = 23.1 Hz), the difference is 13.6 dB
- For f_c = 10,000 Hz (Δf = 2310 Hz), the difference is 33.6 dB
- Thus, from f_c = 100 Hz to f_c = 10,000 Hz, the divergence equals 20 dB
- Finally, 10 log (2310 / 23.1) = 20 dB

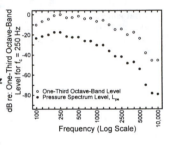

Ch6-94

CHAPTER 7

DISTORTION

Ch7-1

Preamble

- Deliver sound wave (or electrical signal) to a system

- If the system reproduces the waveform <u>faithfully</u>, the signal is <u>undistorted</u>

- If the shape of the waveform is <u>altered</u>, the signal is <u>distorted</u>

Ch7-2

Three Types of Distortion

- Frequency

- Transient

- Amplitude

Ch7-3

FREQUENCY DISTORTION

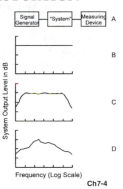

- Panel A: Measurement of amplitude response of a system
  - The input signal must have equal amplitude for all frequencies delivered to the system
- Panel B: No distortion at output of system
  - All frequencies at output have equal amplitude, just as at input

Ch7-4

FREQUENCY DISTORTION

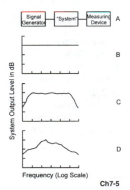

- Note panels C & D
  - All frequencies <u>not</u> reproduced with same amplitude
  - System was frequency selective; filtering occurred
  - Signal underwent <u>frequency distortion</u>

Ch7-5

System Transfer Function

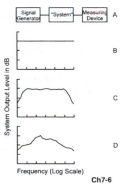

- The three functions in panels B, C, & D describe the <u>system transfer function</u>, or <u>amplitude response</u>, of the system
- The amplitude response reveals evidence of frequency distortion

Ch7-6

93

Linear Systems

- Linear systems alter only the amplitudes and phases of a signal
- They <u>do</u> produce frequency distortion
- "Frequency response" of an audio device might be described as
  - ♦ 100 Hz to 10,000 Hz
  - ♦ Flat ± X dB

Ch7-7

Linear Systems

- Panel A: Input-Output (I/O) function of <u>linear</u> system
  - ♦ As input amplitude increases (e.g., by 5 dB), output amplitude increases <u>proportionally</u> (5 dB)
  - ♦ Output amplitude need not <u>equal</u> input amplitude; the change is a proportional one

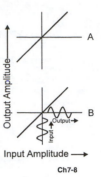

Ch7-8

Linear Systems

- Panel B: The characteristics of the input sine wave are <u>preserved faithfully</u> in output sine wave; Why?
  ☑

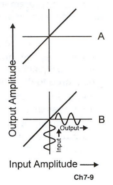

Ch7-9

TRANSIENT DISTORTION

- The amplitude response of a sine wave is <u>not</u> really a line spectrum as shown in panel A; Why?
  - ♦ Its duration is <u>finite</u>

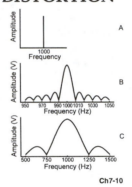

Ch7-10

Effects of Duration on Amplitude Response

- Panel A: Infinite duration
- Panel B: 100 ms tone burst

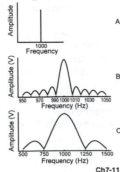

Ch7-11

Effects of Duration on Amplitude Response

- ♦ Energy spread to surrounding frequencies, and amplitude spectrum is <u>continuous</u>
- ♦ Nulls at <u>integer multiples of reciprocal of duration</u> (100 ms)
  - \>> 1/.1 = +/- 10 Hz
  - \>> 2/.1 = +/- 20 Hz
  - \>> 3/.1 = +/- 30 Hz, etc.

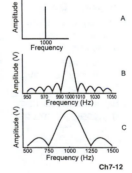

Ch7-12

Effects of Duration on Amplitude Response

- Panel C: Duration shortened from 100 ms to 4 ms
  - 1 / .004 = +/- 250 Hz
  - 2 / .004 = +/- 500 Hz
  - 3 / .004 = +/- 750 Hz, etc
- Thus, width of each <u>lobe</u> is inversely proportional to duration

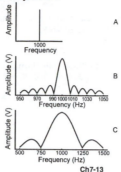

Ch7-13

Effects of Rise-Decay Time on Amplitude Response

- Amplitude rises over time from zero to max, and falls over time from max to zero
- Panel A shows <u>amplitude envelope</u> in the time domain
- Panel B shows <u>amplitude spectrum</u> in the frequency domain

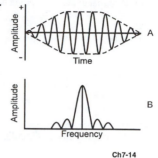

Ch7-14

Effects of Rise-Decay Time on Amplitude Response

- Panel B
  - Energy spread to other frequencies: <u>Continuous spectrum</u>
  - Initiation & termination of signal produces <u>transients</u>

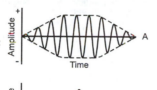

Ch7-15

Effects of Rise-Decay Time on Amplitude Response

- The longer the rise-fall time, the less the transient distortion
- ANSI S3.6-1989
  - Time from -20 dB to -1 dB shall not be less than 20 ms

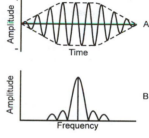

Ch7-16

AMPLITUDE DISTORTION

- Panel A: I/O function for a <u>linear</u> system, compared with
- Panel B: I/O function for a <u>nonlinear</u> system
- Panel C: As input amplitude to <u>linear</u> system (from panel A) changes, output amplitude changes proportionally; <u>no</u> distortion

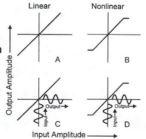

Ch7-17

AMPLITUDE DISTORTION

- Panel D: Input amplitudes do not exceed <u>limits of linearity</u> of nonlinear system; changes in output amplitude still are <u>proportional</u> to changes in input amplitude; <u>no</u> distortion

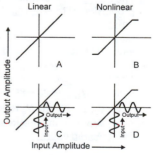

Ch7-18

AMPLITUDE DISTORTION

- Panel A: Do some of the instantaneous amplitudes of the input signal exceed the limits of linearity of the system?
  ☑
- What is the result?
  ☑

- Panel B: more severe peak clipping; more severe distortion

Input Amplitude⟶
Ch7-19

AMPLITUDE DISTORTION

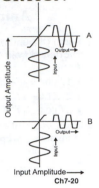

- The distortion is called <u>amplitude distortion</u>; Why?
  ☑

- Amplitude distortion is also called <u>nonlinear distortion</u>; Why?
  ☑

Input Amplitude⟶
Ch7-20

Effects of Amplitude, or Nonlinear, Distortion on Amplitude Spectrum

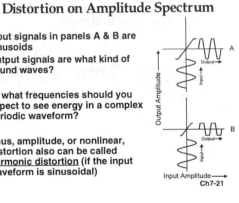

- Input signals in panels A & B are sinusoids
- Output signals are what kind of sound waves?
  ☑
- At what frequencies should you expect to see energy in a complex periodic waveform?
  ☑
- Thus, amplitude, or nonlinear, distortion also can be called <u>harmonic distortion</u> (if the input waveform is sinusoidal)

Input Amplitude⟶
Ch7-21

Effects of Amplitude, or Nonlinear, Distortion on Amplitude Spectrum

- The figure displays the output spectrum from a nonlinear system
- At the input, f = 100 Hz
- At the output, note energy at harmonics of f_0

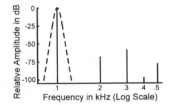

Ch7-22

Percentage Harmonic Distortion

- <u>The concept:</u> Percentage harmonic distortion is proportion of <u>total energy</u> that is <u>undesired energy</u>
- Measure the voltage (V) of the output spectrum with a 1/3-octave filter and voltmeter
- Set f_c of the filter to equal, progressively, the frequency of each harmonic selectively
  - V_2, V_3, V_4, and V_5 reflect <u>undesired energy</u>
  - V_1, V_2, V_3, V_4, and V_5 reflect <u>total energy</u>
- Next, compute the proportion of <u>total energy</u> that is <u>undesired energy</u>

Ch7-23

Calculation

- % = (Undesired Energy / Total Energy) × 100

  - $= \dfrac{f\,(V_2, V_3, V_4.....V_n)}{f\,(V_1, V_2, V_3.....V_n)} \times 100$, where

    >> f is some undefined function

    >> Vs cannot be summed

Ch7-24

Calculation

♦ $= \dfrac{f'\,(V_2^2 + V_3^2 + V_4^2 + \ldots V_n^2)}{f'\,(V_1^2 + V_2^2 + V_3^2 + \ldots V_n^2)} \times 100$

>> Vs are squared ($W \propto V^2$) so summing now permissible

♦ $= \dfrac{\sqrt{(V_2^2 + V_3^2 + V_4^2 + \ldots + V_n^2)}}{\sqrt{(V_1^2 + V_2^2 + V_3^2 + \ldots + V_n^2)}} \times 100$

>> Return to voltages by taking square root of sum ($V \propto \sqrt{W}$)

Ch7-25

Approximate Percentage Harmonic Distortion

● $\% = \dfrac{\sqrt{V_2^2 + V_3^2 + V_4^2 + \ldots + V_n^2}}{\sqrt{V_1^2}} \times 100$

● How do we justify the approximation?

● Most of total energy in denominator comes from f_0 (V_1)

● Contribution of V_2, V_3, V_4, and V_5 is usually negligible

Ch7-26

Amplitude Response and Dynamic Range

● Panel A: I/O functions for several driving frequencies from .1 kHz to 10 kHz

  ♦ On each I/O function, location of the filled dot identifies point of maximum permissible harmonic distortion

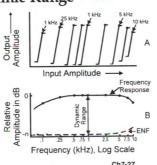

Ch7-27

Amplitude Response and Dynamic Range

● Panel B: The dots from I/O functions are connected and redrawn in the frequency domain to form the upper curve

  ♦ That defines the amplitude response of the system

  ♦ Electrical noise floor (ENF) of system is shown by lower curve

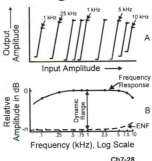

Ch7-28

Amplitude Response and Dynamic Range

● Dynamic range is distance in decibels from ENF to amplitude response at maximum

● Does ENF vary with frequency?
  ☑

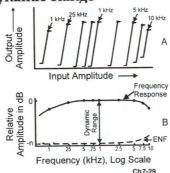

Ch7-29

Intermodulation Distortion

● Driving signal is complex

● Experience nonlinear distortion

● Result called <u>intermodulation distortion</u>

Ch7-30

Intermodulation Distortion

- Suppose <u>input signal</u> has two frequency components
  - ◆ $f_1 = 100$ Hz
  - ◆ $f_2 = 110$ Hz
- Frequency components of <u>output signal</u> include two types of distortion products:
  - ◆ Harmonics
  - ◆ Combination Tones
    - \>> Difference tones
    - \>> Summation tones

Ch7-31

Intermodulation Distortion

- 1. Harmonics of each frequency component
  - ◆ $1f_1 = 100$ Hz & $1f_2 = 110$ Hz
  - ◆ $2f_1 = 200$ Hz & $2f_2 = 220$ Hz
  - ◆ $3f_1 = 300$ Hz & $3f_2 = 330$ Hz, etc.

Table 7-2. Examples of harmonics and combination tones produced for a complex wave with two frequency components, $f_1 = 100$ Hz and $f_2 = 110$ Hz

HARMONICS OF		COMBINATION TONES	
f_1	f_2	Difference Tones	Summation Tones
$\lvert 1f_1 + 0f_2 \rvert = 100$	$\lvert 0f_1 + 1f_2 \rvert = 110$	$\lvert 1f_1 - 1f_2 \rvert = 10$	$\lvert 1f_1 + 1f_2 \rvert = 210$
$\lvert 2f_1 + 0f_2 \rvert = 200$	$\lvert 0f_1 + 2f_2 \rvert = 220$	$\lvert 2f_1 - 1f_2 \rvert = 90$	$\lvert 2f_1 + 1f_2 \rvert = 310$
$\lvert 3f_1 + 0f_2 \rvert = 300$	$\lvert 0f_1 + 3f_2 \rvert = 330$	$\lvert 3f_1 - 1f_2 \rvert = 190$	$\lvert 3f_1 + 1f_2 \rvert = 410$
etc.	etc.	etc.	etc.

Intermodulation Distortion

- 2. <u>Difference</u> tones:
  - ◆ $\lvert 1f_1 - f_2 \rvert = 10$ Hz
  - ◆ $\lvert 2f_1 - f_2 \rvert = 90$ Hz
  - ◆ $\lvert 3f_1 - f_2 \rvert = 190$ Hz, etc.

Table 7-2. Examples of harmonics and combination tones produced for a complex wave with two frequency components, $f_1 = 100$ Hz and $f_2 = 110$ Hz

HARMONICS OF		COMBINATION TONES	
f_1	f_2	Difference Tones	Summation Tones
$\lvert 1f_1 + 0f_2 \rvert = 100$	$\lvert 0f_1 + 1f_2 \rvert = 110$	$\lvert 1f_1 - 1f_2 \rvert = 10$	$\lvert 1f_1 + 1f_2 \rvert = 210$
$\lvert 2f_1 + 0f_2 \rvert = 200$	$\lvert 0f_1 + 2f_2 \rvert = 220$	$\lvert 2f_1 - 1f_2 \rvert = 90$	$\lvert 2f_1 + 1f_2 \rvert = 310$
$\lvert 3f_1 + 0f_2 \rvert = 300$	$\lvert 0f_1 + 3f_2 \rvert = 330$	$\lvert 3f_1 - 1f_2 \rvert = 190$	$\lvert 3f_1 + 1f_2 \rvert = 410$
etc.	etc.	etc.	etc.

Intermodulation Distortion

- 3. <u>Summation</u> tones:
  - ◆ $1f_1 + f_2 = 210$ Hz
  - ◆ $2f_1 + f_2 = 310$ Hz
  - ◆ $3f_1 + f_2 = 410$ Hz, etc.

Table 7-2. Examples of harmonics and combination tones produced for a complex wave with two frequency components, $f_1 = 100$ Hz and $f_2 = 110$ Hz

HARMONICS OF		COMBINATION TONES	
f_1	f_2	Difference Tones	Summation Tones
$\lvert 1f_1 + 0f_2 \rvert = 100$	$\lvert 0f_1 + 1f_2 \rvert = 110$	$\lvert 1f_1 - 1f_2 \rvert = 10$	$\lvert 1f_1 + 1f_2 \rvert = 210$
$\lvert 2f_1 + 0f_2 \rvert = 200$	$\lvert 0f_1 + 2f_2 \rvert = 220$	$\lvert 2f_1 - 1f_2 \rvert = 90$	$\lvert 2f_1 + 1f_2 \rvert = 310$
$\lvert 3f_1 + 0f_2 \rvert = 300$	$\lvert 0f_1 + 3f_2 \rvert = 330$	$\lvert 3f_1 - 1f_2 \rvert = 190$	$\lvert 3f_1 + 1f_2 \rvert = 410$
etc.	etc.	etc.	etc.

Combination Tones

- Equation 7.3 defines frequencies of all harmonics, difference tones, and summation tones
  - ◆ $mf_1 \pm nf_2$, where
  - ◆ m and n are assigned all integer values

Ch7-35

CHAPTER 8

SOUND TRANSMISSION

Ch8-1

Preamble

- Sound fades away over distance
- Sound fades away over time
- Sound waves encounter obstacles

Ch8-2

ATTENUATION OF SOUND INTENSITY OVER DISTANCE

- When sound is propagated in a free, unbounded medium (a medium with no obstacles to affect wave propagation), intensity decreases in a lawful way
- This is called the <u>inverse square law</u>
- Imagine sound produced by a point source in a free, unbounded medium
  - ♦ A longitudinal wave is propagated through the medium

Ch8-3

Spherical Waves

- Compressions form a "spherical shell," which is called a <u>wave front</u>
  - ♦ Wave front moves outward from source to A, B, C, etc.
  - ♦ How does wave front at C differ from wave fronts at B and A? Beyond C?
  - ☑

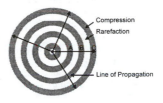

Compression
Rarefaction

Line of Propagation

Ch8-4

Plane Waves

- At some distance from source the <u>spherical</u> wave front becomes a <u>plane wave front</u>: Why?
- ☑

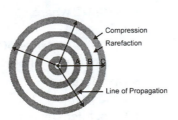

Compression
Rarefaction

Line of Propagation

Ch8-5

Plane Waves

- Sine waves are <u>spherical</u>, or <u>plane progressive</u>, <u>waves</u> in a free, unbounded medium
  - ♦ Imagine a soap bubble becoming progressively larger; surface of bubble represents a wave front

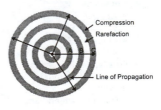

Compression
Rarefaction

Line of Propagation

Ch8-6

99

THE INVERSE SQUARE LAW

- From A to B to C, <u>energy</u> is dissipated over a larger & larger surface area
- <u>Power</u> is energy / s
  - ♦ Therefore, same amount of power is dissipated over larger and larger surface areas.

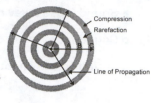

Compression
Rarefaction

Line of Propagation

Ch8-7

THE INVERSE SQUARE LAW

- <u>Intensity</u> is energy / s / m^2
- If power remains constant, but surface area increases, what happens to intensity? ☑
- Analogous to a constant force being exerted on a larger & larger area
  - ♦ Pressure (F / A) decreases

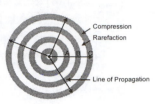

Compression
Rarefaction

Line of Propagation

Ch8-8

Intensity

- Place eye at point source and look outward at areas bounded by four lines of propagation
  - ♦ Intensity at 2X is 1 / 4 that at X
  - ♦ At 4X it is 1 / 4 that at 2X
  - ♦ and so on
- Intensity decreases lawfully -- the <u>inverse square law</u>. Why?
  - ♦ Intensity varies <u>inversely</u> with the <u>square</u> of the distance

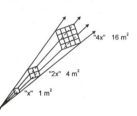

"4x" 16 m^2

"2x" 4 m^2

"x" 1 m^2

Ch8-9

Intensity

- Area of sphere
  - ♦ A = 4πr^2
- Thus,
  - ♦ At 1m, A = 12.6 m^2 (4π1^2)
  - ♦ At 2m, A = 50.3 m^2 (4π2^2)
  - ♦ At 4m, A = 201.1 m^2 (4π4^2)

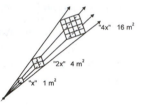

"4x" 16 m^2

"2x" 4 m^2

"x" 1 m^2

Ch8-10

Intensity

- Moreover,
  - ♦ At 2m, 50.3 = 12.6^2
  - ♦ At 4m, 201.1 = 50.3^2
- Finally, if A increases, energy / s / m^2 must decrease
  - ♦ Between 1m and 2m, A increases by 4:1
  - ♦ ∴ I must decrease--1:4

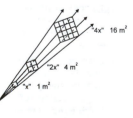

"4x" 16 m^2

"2x" 4 m^2

"x" 1 m^2

Ch8-11

THE INVERSE SQUARE LAW

- I ∝ 1 / D^2, where
  - ♦ D = d$_i$ / d$_r$
    - >> d$_i$ is distance of interest, &
    - >> d$_r$ is reference distance
- Therefore:
  - ♦ I ∝ 1 / (d$_i$ / d$_r$)^2
- Thus, intensity is <u>inversely</u> proportional to the <u>square</u> of the ratio of two distances, d$_i$ and d$_r$

Ch8-12

The Inverse Square Law and Decibels

- **How could we express the decrease in decibels?**
- **dB = 10 $\log_{10}$ 1 / $(d_i / d_r)^2$**
    - ♦ **= - 10 $\log_{10}$ $(d_i / d_r)^2$ Why?**
      ☑
    - ♦ **= - 20 $\log_{10}$ (d_i / d_r) Why?**
      ☑

Ch8-13

The Inverse Square Law and Decibels

- **Compare intensity at 2X with X: How many dB?**
  ☑

- **Compare intensity at 4X with 2X: How many dB?**
  ☑

- **Compare intensity at 4X with X: How many dB?**
  ☑

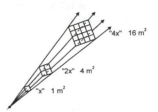

Ch8-14

Sample Problems

1. **SPL = 90 dB at distance of 100 m from source. By how much is SPL <u>decreased</u> at 200 m?**
   ☑

2. **What is <u>SPL</u> at 200 m?**
   ☑

Ch8-15

Sample Problems

3. **SPL = 100 dB at 100 m from source. By how much is SPL decreased at 200 m?**
   ☑

4. **SPL = 80 dB at 100 m. What is <u>SPL</u> at 750 m?**
   ☑
   ☑

Ch8-16

Sample Problems

5. **SPL of gunshot is 110 dB at 0.5 miles. Should shot be heard at 8,192 miles if threshold for hearing is 20 dB SPL?**
   ☑
   ☑
   ☑
   ☑

Ch8-17

THE INVERSE SQUARE LAW

- **Inverse square law only holds strictly in free, unbounded medium with no obstacles**
- **If sound wave encounters obstacle, it will be:**
    - ♦ **reflected,**
    - ♦ **refracted,**
    - ♦ **diffracted, or**
    - ♦ **absorbed**
- **Will inverse square law then hold strictly?**
  ☑

Ch8-18

THE INVERSE SQUARE LAW

- In what ways will it differ for reflection and absorption?
  ☑

  ☑

Ch8-19

REFLECTION

- Animation F8-3
- Angle of reflected path to the perpendicular equals angle of the incident path to the perpendicular

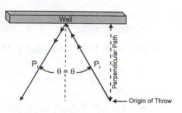

Ch8-20

Reflection of Sound Waves

- Animation F8-4
- Spherical wave fronts generated by point source at s move from right to left -- encounter plane obstacle
- Obstacle offers large acoustic impedance
- A ray is a line perpendicular to the wave front

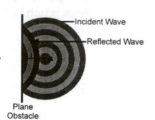

Ch8-21

Reflection of Sound Waves

- With no obstacle, wave fronts would continue on toward s'
- Because of obstacle, sound wave is reflected back toward source with no change in speed of propagation
- Angles of the reflected rays to the perpendicular equal angles of incident rays to the perpendicular

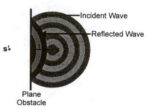

Ch8-22

Reflection of Sound Waves

- Energy is retained in medium and inverse square law does not hold
- Is the decrease in intensity < or > the law would predict?
  ☑

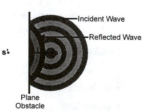

Ch8-23

Reflection From Plane Surfaces

- Angles of reflected rays equal angles of incident rays to perpendicular
  ♦ 45° in panel A
  ♦ 30° in panel B
- Under what circumstance will a ray be reflected back on itself toward source?
  ☑

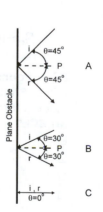

Ch8-24

Reflection From Convex Surfaces

- Animation F8-6
- Panel A: Obstacle surface is <u>convex</u> toward source of sound
  - ♦ Two incident rays are shown, i_1, i_2
- Reflected rays <u>diverge</u>; sound energy is <u>scattered</u>
- Intensity of reflected wave?
  ☑

- Example?
  ☑

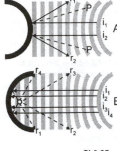

Ch8-25

Reflection From Concave Surfaces

- Panel B: Obstacle surface is <u>concave</u> toward source of sound
  - ♦ Four incident rays are shown
- Reflected waves <u>converge</u>; sound energy is "collected" or <u>concentrated</u>
- Rays converge at focal point; energy density (intensity) is maximal
- Intensity of reflected wave?
  ☑
- Example?
  ☑

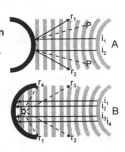

Ch8-26

Sound Wave Reflection (Summary)

- Regardless of whether the obstacle surface is plane, convex, or concave

- The angles of reflected rays to the perpendicular equal the angles of incident rays to the perpendicular

Ch8-27

Echoes, Reverberation, and Reverberation Time

- Reflected waves often are called echoes or reverberating waves
  - ♦ Contrast reverberant rooms with anechoic rooms
    - >> Reverberant: rooms with hard surfaces to maximize reflections
    - >> Anechoic: rooms with absorbing surfaces to minimize reflections

Ch8-28

Echoes, Reverberation, and Reverberation Time

- Reverberation Time
  - ♦ Time required for sound energy to decay by 60 dB (T_{60})
  - ♦ Volcanic explosion in Krakatoa in East Indies (1883) -- from barometric records speed of sound estimated at 320 m/s

Ch8-29

Standing Waves

- Occur when two progressive waves, incident and reflected, of same frequency & amplitude, travel in opposite directions in or along medium
- Consider standing waves for transverse waves separate from those for longitudinal waves
- Will conclude by relating standing waves to resonant frequencies of strings and tubes

Ch8-30

Transverse Wave Motion and Standing Waves

- Animation F8-7
- **Panel A:** String stretched with some fixed tension; dots painted at equal intervals
- **Panel B:** Source of sound causes one sound wave (dashed) to travel from left to right
- A second source causes a second wave (solid) to travel from right to left

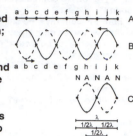

Ch8-31

Transverse Wave Motion and Standing Waves

- Points b, d, f, h, & j move alternately up and down: called displacement <u>antinodes</u> -- points of maximum vibration
- Points a, c, e, g, i, & k remain stationary: called displacement <u>nodes</u> -- points of no vibration

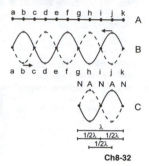

Ch8-32

Transverse Wave Motion and Standing Waves

- <u>Loops</u> are formed between adjacent nodes
- **Panel C:** one cycle of each transverse wave:
  - Two <u>loops</u> are formed
- Distance between two nodes, or between two antinodes, <u>corresponds to one-half wavelength</u>

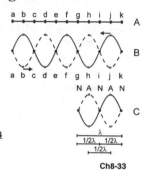

Ch8-33

Transverse Wave Motion and Standing Waves

- Each wave is moving -- one from left to right, the other from right to left -- but the resultant wave is stationary
  - A standing wave

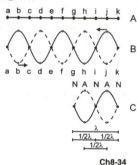

Ch8-34

Longitudinal Wave Motion and Standing Waves

- **Panel A:** Air-filled tube open at one end and closed at the other end
  - Incident waves travel from L-R; will be reflected by closed end
  - Reflected waves travel from R-L
  - Two waves will interact along length of tube

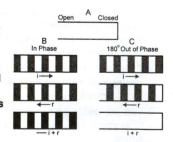

Ch8-35

Longitudinal Wave Motion and Standing Waves

- **Panel B:** Incident & reflected waves are <u>in phase</u>: What happens? ☑

- **Panel C:** Incident & reflected waves are <u>out of phase</u>: What happens? ☑

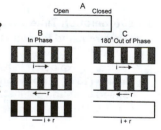

Ch8-36

Longitudinal Wave Motion and Standing Waves

- The two waves are moving <u>in</u> and <u>out</u> of phase over time
  - ♦ Each wave is traveling, but
  - ♦ Resultant wave is <u>stationary</u>
- At certain locations, dependent on L and f, they are always <u>in phase</u> -- at others, they are always <u>out of phase</u>

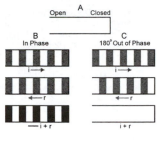

Ch8-37

Longitudinal Wave Motion and Standing Waves

- Interaction of incident and reflected waves
  - ♦ Dotted Line: Incident R-L
  - ♦ Dashed Line: Reflected L-R
  - ♦ Blue line: Resultant
- Resultant is point-by-point summation of i and r

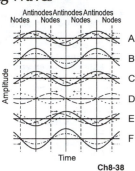

Ch8-38

Longitudinal Wave Motion and Standing Waves

- Suppose f = 125 Hz; T = ?
- ☑
- Each panel = 1 ms interval, or 1/8 of a period

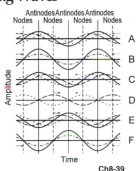

Ch8-39

Longitudinal Wave Motion and Standing Waves

- Solid vertical lines positioned on <u>antinodes</u>
  - ♦ A: partially in phase -- partial reinforcement
  - ♦ B: in phase -- maximal reinforcement
  - ♦ C: same as A
  - ♦ D: 180° out of phase -- cancellation
  - ♦ E: same as C, but opposite
  - ♦ F: same as B, but opposite

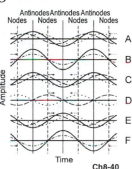

Ch8-40

Longitudinal Wave Motion and Standing Waves

- Dashed vertical lines positioned on <u>nodes</u>
- What happens at nodal point over time from A to F?
  - ☑
  - ☑

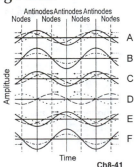

Ch8-41

Standing Waves and Resonant Frequencies

- Tube open at one end; closed at other
- Panel A: Displacement pattern of air mass from 0° (equilibrium), to 90° (x_{max}), to 180°, to 270°, & to 0°: <u>one cycle</u>
  - ♦ Two dashed lines trace maximum displacement (x_{max} envelope) patterns at 90° & 270° along length of tube

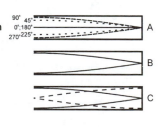

Ch8-42

Standing Waves and Resonant Frequencies

- Panel B: Displacement envelope from panel A
  - ◆ Displacement <u>node</u>: Closed end
  - ◆ Displacement <u>antinode</u>: Open end
- Panel C: Comparison of displacement and pressure nodes & antinodes
  - ◆ Pressure <u>node</u>: Open end
  - ◆ Pressure <u>antinode</u>: Closed end

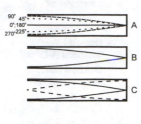

Ch8-43

Standing Waves and Resonant Frequencies

- Panel B: Displacement envelope
  - ◆ One node, one antinode, & 1/2 of one loop
  - ◆ Thus, standing wave created with $\lambda = 1/4$ length (L) of tube
    - $>> \lambda = s/f$
    - $>> f = s/\lambda$

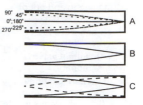

Ch8-44

Standing Waves and Resonant Frequencies

- ◆ For open-closed tube
  - $>> F_1 = 1s/4L$ (F_1 is first, or lowest, of series of resonances)
  - $>>$ other resonances will be <u>odd</u> integer multiples of F_1

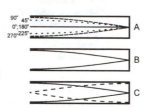

Ch8-45

Standing Waves and Resonant Frequencies

- Panel A: Lowest resonant frequency-- $F_1 = 1s/4L$
- Panel B: F_2
  - ◆ 2 nodes, 2 antinodes, and 1 1/2 loops
    - $>> 1$ loop $= 1/4\lambda$
    - $>> 1\ 1/2$ loops $= 3/4\lambda$
  - ◆ $F_2 = 3s/4L$

A $\left(F_1 = \frac{1s}{4L}\right)$

B $\left(F_2 = \frac{3s}{4L}\right)$

C $\left(F_3 = \frac{5s}{4L}\right)$

Ch8-46

Standing Waves and Resonant Frequencies

- Panel C: F_3
  - ◆ 3 nodes, 3 antinodes, and 2 1/2 loops
    - $>> 1$ loop $= 1/4\lambda$
    - $>> 2\ 1/2$ loops $= 5/4\lambda$
  - ◆ $F_3 = ?$
    - ☑

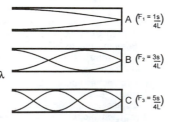

A $\left(F_1 = \frac{1s}{4L}\right)$

B $\left(F_2 = \frac{3s}{4L}\right)$

C $\left(F_3 = \frac{5s}{4L}\right)$

Ch8-47

Sample Computations

- $L = .17\ m; s = 340\ m/s$
- $F_1 = ?$
  - ☑
- $F_2 = ?$
  - ☑
- $F_3 = ?$
  - ☑
- Higher resonances are <u>odd</u> integer multiples of F_1
  - ◆ $F_2 = 3\ F_1$
  - ◆ $F_3 = 5\ F_1$

Ch8-48

Standing Waves and Resonant Frequencies

- What happens to F_1, F_2, and F_3 if L is shortened?

  ☑

  ☑

- Equation 8.9

  - $F_n = [(2n) -1]s/4L$, where

  - $n = n^{th}$ resonance

Standing Waves and Resonant Frequencies

- Why not odd <u>and</u> even integer multiples of F_1?
  - Displacement node <u>must</u> be at closed end
  - Displacement antinode <u>must</u> be at open end
- Proof
  - If F_1 corresponds to 1/4 λ and 1/2 loop
  - $2F_1$ corresponds to 1/2 λ and 1 loop
  - To fit 1 loop into tube requires either
    - \>> 2 antinodes and 1 node, or
    - \>> 1 antinode and 2 nodes
  - neither is possible

Standing Waves and Resonant Frequencies

- Panel A: Tube open at both ends
  - Displacement antinodes at open ends
  - Displacement node in middle
- Panel B: Tube closed at both ends
  - Displacement nodes at both ends
  - Displacement antinode in middle

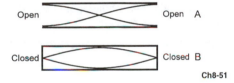

Standing Waves and Resonant Frequencies

- Panels A <u>and</u> B
  - 1 loop; 1/2 λ
  - $F_1 = 1s/2L$
  - $F_n = ns/2L$
  - Higher resonances are <u>odd and even</u> integer multiples of F_1

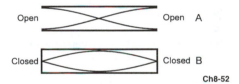

Sample Computations

- $L = .17$ m; $s = 340$ m/s
- $F_1 = ?$

  ☑

- $F_2 = ?$

  ☑

- $F_3 = ?$

  ☑

- Higher resonances are <u>odd and even</u> integer multiples of F_1

Vibration of Strings

- Equation 2.10 from Chapter 2
  - $f = 1/2L(\sqrt{t/m})$
- That solves for <u>lowest</u> of a series of frequencies, f_0
- String also vibrates at harmonics of f_0
- Harmonics are <u>odd and even</u> integer multiples of f_0
- String is fixed at both ends
  - Analogous to tube closed at both ends
  - Displacement node at each end
  - Displacement antinode midway

Vibration of Strings

- **Panel A:** Stretched string attached to two pegs
- **Panel B:** Displacement pattern over time
  - ◆ 1 loop; 1/2 λ
  - ◆ $f_0 = 1s/2L$, where
    - >> s = speed of sound
      $(s = \sqrt{t/m})$
    - >> L = length

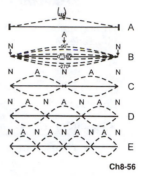

Ch8-55

Vibration of Strings

- **Panels C, D, & E**
  - ◆ 2 loops; 3 loops; & 4 loops
  - ◆ 1λ; 1 1/2 λ; 2λ
- $f_n = ns/2L$, where n (coefficients) are integers
- Higher harmonics are <u>odd</u> and <u>even</u> integer multiples (harmonics) of f_0

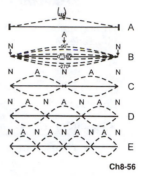

Ch8-56

Sample Computations

- s = 420 m/s; L = .93 m
- What is f_0?
  - ☑
- What are fs of next three harmonics?
  - ☑
  - ☑
  - ☑
- Harmonics are <u>odd</u> and <u>even</u> integer multiples of f_0

Ch8-57

REFRACTION

- **Recall:** When a wave encounters an obstacle offering large impedance, the wave is reflected with <u>no change in speed of propagation</u>

- Now consider the case in which a wave moves to another medium, or encounters a change in the medium

- Speed of propagation changes and rays are bent

Ch8-58

REFRACTION

- Light waves travel from air (M_1) to water (M_2)
- $s_{M_1} > s_{M_2}$
- Image of stick is bent because of change in speed (s) of propagation: Snell's Law
- Refraction of sound waves: Bending of wave fronts due to change in speed of propagation

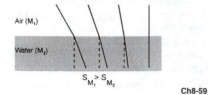

Air (M_1)

Water (M_2)

$S_{M_1} > S_{M_2}$

Ch8-59

Sound Traveling With and Against Wind

- **Animation F8-15**
- **Panel A:** Sound travels L to R: No wind
  - ◆ Wave fronts are not bent
- **Panel B:** Wind speed shown as a vector quantity
  - ◆ What is shown?
    - ☑

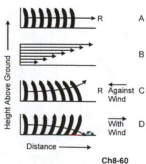

Ch8-60

Sound Traveling With and Against Wind

- Panel C: Sound travels <u>against</u> wind
  - ◆ What happens to wave fronts?
    - ☑
- Panel D: Sound travels <u>with</u> wind
  - ◆ What happens?
    - ☑
- Sound travels farther <u>with</u> wind

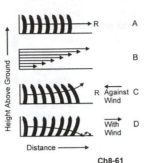

Ch8-61

Sound Traveling in Early Morning vs. Midday

- Animation F8-16
- Panel A: Early morning
  - ◆ Warmer air is higher
  - ◆ Warmer air has less density
  - ◆ Less density -- increased speed $s = \sqrt{E/\rho}$
  - ◆ Wave fronts refracted downward, reflected upward, etc.

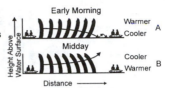

Ch8-62

Sound Traveling in Early Morning vs. Midday

- Panel B: Midday
  - ◆ Warmer air is lower
  - ◆ What happens differently?
    - ☑

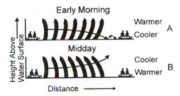

Ch8-63

Reflected by Water?

- $Z_{water} > Z_{air}$
- 0.1% of incident energy penetrates water surface
- 99.9% reflected by water
- dB attenuation of wave from air to water?
  - ◆ $dB = 10 \log_{10} (I_x / I_r) = 10 \log_{10} (10^{-3} / 10^0)$
    $= -30$ dB

Ch8-64

Attenuation in Air?

- 99.9% reflected by water
- How much is sound wave in air attenuated?
  - ☑

Ch8-65

DIFFRACTION

- What happens when water wave encounters a diving raft?
  - ◆ The wave <u>bends</u> around obstacle and reforms
  - ◆ This is called <u>diffraction</u>

Ch8-66

Diffraction

- Panel A: plane progressive wave moving L-R
- Wave encounters barrier
  - ◆ Some energy reflected back
  - ◆ Wave fronts scatter, or bend, around obstacle
  - ◆ Wave fronts then reform and continue as plane wave fronts

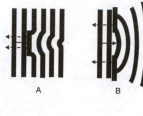

Ch8-67

Diffraction

- Panel B: Wave fronts encounter opening in wall
  - ◆ Some energy reflected back
  - ◆ Portions of wave fronts pass through and then reform as plane waves

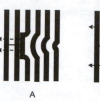

Ch8-68

ABSORPTION

- Opposition to sound transmission will exist at <u>any boundary</u> where impedances differ

- If impedance is infinite, intensity of reflected wave will equal intensity of incident wave

  - ◆ $I_r = I_i$

Ch8-69

Absorption

- If impedance is not infinite, some sound energy will be <u>absorbed</u> by new medium

- Intensity of reflected wave will be less than intensity of incident wave

  - ◆ $I_r < I_i$

Ch8-70

Absorption Coefficient

- Magnitude of absorption given by absorption coefficient, α
- α is the proportion of energy in incident wave absorbed by material
- $\alpha = I_a / I_i$, where
  - ◆ I_a = energy absorbed and
  - ◆ I_i = energy of incident wave
- Air to water
  - ◆ 0.1% absorbed
  - ◆ 99.9% reflected

Ch8-71

Absorption

- Suppose SPL_i = 80 dB

  - ◆ I_i = 10^{-4} watt/m^2

- Attenuate 30 dB

  - ◆ I_a = 10^{-7} watt/m^2

  - ◆ $I_a / I_i = 10^{-7} / 10^{-4} = 10^{-3}$

  - ◆ α = .001

Ch8-72

Absorption

- If SPL_i = 80 dB, and .1% is absorbed, what is SPL of sound wave retained in medium?

☑

☑

☑

☑

Absorption

- Does "α" vary with intensity of incident wave; I_i ?

☑

☑

Sound-Treated Rooms

- <u>Anechoic rooms</u> have high absorption coefficient
  - ◆ Fiberglass wedges are absorbing material
- Sound isolated rooms
  - ◆ Designed to reduce sound transmission through walls
  - ◆ Reasonably high absorption coefficient

Absorption and Reflection

- Absorption is inversely proportional to reflection

- Thus, as absorption coefficient increases, reflection & reverberation time decrease

Absorption and Reflection

- Absorption coefficient, α, varies with frequency and with nature of materials

	Frequency in kHz					
	.125	.25	.5	1	2	4
Vinyl tile on concrete	.02	.03	.03	.03	.03	.02
Painted concrete block	.1	.1	.1	.1	.1	.1
Window glass	.3	.2	.2	.1	.1	.05
Plaster on lath	.2	.2	.1	.1	.05	.1
Unpainted concrete block	.4	.4	.3	.3	.4	.3
Thick carpet on concrete	.02	.06	.15	.4	.6	.6
Thick carpet on felt pad	.1	.3	.4	.5	.6	.7
Occupied upholstered seating	.4	.6	.8	.9	.9	.9

Total Absorption

- <u>Total</u> absorption in a room depends on
  - ◆ Absorption coefficients of materials in room and
  - ◆ Room volume
- Quantified by <u>absorption units</u>
  - ◆ Sabine (fps)
  - ◆ Metric sabine (MKS)
- Total absorption for opening of 1 m^2 (MKS)
- Large, bare room with open window 1 m^2
  - ◆ α of window = 1.0 (100% absorption)

Absorption and Reflection

- Assume six surfaces of room absorb equally
- Theoretical reverberation time, T_{60}:
  - $T_{60} \propto V$ (volume of room)
  - $T_{60} \propto 1/A$ (area of opening)
  - $T_{60} = k \, (V/A)$
    >>$k = .049$ (fps)
    >>$k = .161$ (MKS)
- If V increases by some factor, x,
  - T_{60} <u>increases</u> by x
  - Sound energy <u>retained</u> in room for longer time
- If A increases by some factor, x,
  - T_{60} <u>decreases</u> by x
  - Sound energy <u>escapes</u> room more quickly

Ch8-79

Total Absorption (A´)

- $A´ = S_1 \alpha_1 + S_2 \alpha_2 + \ldots + S_n \alpha_n$
  - S = surface area
  - α = absorption coefficient of surface (S_n)
- Thus, A´, for multiple absorbing surfaces equals sum of the total absorption ($S_n \alpha_n$) of the individual surfaces

Ch8-80

Sample Computation (f = 500 Hz)

	Dimensions (m)	S	α	A
Side wall	3×20	60	.10	6.0
Side wall	3×20	60	.10	6.0
End wall	3×12	36	.10	3.6
End wall	3×12	36	.40	14.4
Floor	12×20	240	.40	96.0
Ceiling	12×20	240	.10	24.0

A´ = 150.0 Ch8-81

Sample Computation (f = 500 Hz)

- $A´ = 150$
- $V = (3 \times 12 \times 20) = 720 \ m^3$
- $T_{60} = k \, (V/A´)$

  $= .161 \, (720 / 150)$

  $= .77 \ s$

  $= 770 \ ms$

Ch8-82

Optimal T_{60}

- Speech in conference room
  - 400 - 800 ms
- Chamber music
  - 900 - 1400 ms
- Organ music
  - 1500 - 2400 ms
- T_{60} varies with V and f

Ch8-83

Absorption and Diffraction

- Air medium itself absorbs sound energy above 1000 Hz
- Example of fog horn vs. whistle for ships at sea
  - Foggy conditions
  - Air contains water droplets with small size re: λ of foghorn sound
  - Sound energy diffracted
  - Whistle with high f
    >> short λ
    >> absorption

Ch8-84

OTHER PHENOMENA IN SOUND TRANSMISSION

- 1. Beats
- 2. Doppler Effect
- 3. Sonic Booms

Ch8-85

1. Beats

- Two people walking at different rates:
    - One at 60 steps / min
    - One at 64 steps / min
- Moving in and out of step (in and out of phase)
- They will be "in step" 4 times / min (64 - 60) and "out of step" 4 times / min

Ch8-86

Beats

- Same principle applies to sine waves of different frequency in same medium
- Because frequencies differ, they will move <u>in and out of phase</u>

Ch8-87

Beats (Example)

- f_1 = 496 Hz
- f_2 = 500 Hz
- In phase 4 times per s and <u>reinforce each other</u>
    - intensity increases
- Out of phase 4 times per s and <u>interfere with each other</u>
    - intensity decreases

Ch8-88

Example

- Result
    - Periodic increases & decreases in <u>amplitude</u>; called <u>beats</u>
    - <u>Beat frequency</u>: The rate at which changes in <u>amplitude</u> occur
- <u>Beat frequency</u> = f_2 - f_1
    - 500 - 496 = 4 Hz
- <u>Pitch</u> corresponds to: $(f_2 + f_1)$ / 2
    - (500 + 496) / 2 = 498 Hz

Ch8-89

Another Example

- Panel A: f_1 = 50 Hz
- Panel B: f_2 = 55 Hz
- Panel C: resultant wave
    - At t = 0 and 200 ms,
    >> in phase
    >> constructive interference
    >> intensity increases

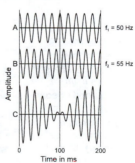

Ch8-90

Another Example

♦ At t = 100 ms,

>> 180° out of phase

>> destructive interference

>> cancellation

>> intensity is momentarily zero

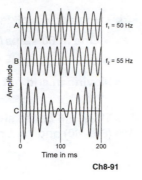

Ch8-91

Example

● Why 200 ms interval between intensity maxima?

● What is beat frequency?

☑

● What is beat period?

☑

● To what frequency does pitch correspond?

☑

Ch8-92

2. The Doppler Effect

● Strike tuning fork of 250 Hz

♦ Air particles displaced at rate of 250 Hz

♦ Disturbance propagated at rate of 340 m/s (speed of sound)

● That is true when <u>source and receiver are stationary</u>

Ch8-93

The Doppler Effect

● If <u>source</u> moves <u>toward</u> observer, pitch rises

● If source moves <u>away</u> from observer, pitch falls

● Called the <u>Doppler effect</u>

Ch8-94

The Doppler Effect

● A is location of <u>moving source</u>

● C is location of <u>stationary receiver</u> (340 m from A)

● s is speed of sound (vector): 340 m/s

● s_s is speed of moving source (vector): 85 m/s

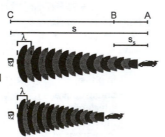

Ch8-95

The Doppler Effect

● Distance AC (340 m) = speed of sound (s = 340 m/s)

● Distance AB (85 m) = speed of moving source (s_s = 85 m/s)

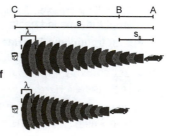

Ch8-96

The Doppler Effect

- A remains stationary
  - ♦ Compressions (& rarefactions) distributed over distance AC after 1 s
- A moves toward C
  - ♦ After 1 s, A moves to B
  - ♦ Same number of compressions crowded into distance BC
- What happens to λ ? ☑
- What happens to f? ☑

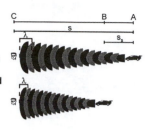

Ch8-97

Another Example

- Frequency   = 400 Hz
- Speed of sound = 340 m/s
- Speed of source = 85 m/s
  - ♦ Altered f   = 533 Hz
  - ♦ As source moves away, f drops from 400 Hz to 320 Hz

Ch8-98

The Equations

- Toward observer
  - ♦ $f' = f(s/s - s_s)$
  - ♦ = 400 (340/340 - 85) = 533 Hz
- Away from observer
  - ♦ $f' = f(s/s + s_s)$
  - ♦ = 400 (340/340 + 85) = 320 Hz

Ch8-99

3. Sonic Booms

- Occur when airplane exceeds speed of sound
- Ratio of speed of airplane to speed of sound is called a <u>Mach number</u>
  - ♦ If airplane speed is 340 m/s, it has achieved Mach 1
  - ♦ At 680 m/s, Mach 2, etc.

Ch8-100

Sonic Booms

- Below Mach 1, airplane is "chasing its own sound wave"
- As plane accelerates, sound waves in front impede flight
  - ♦ More thrust is required
- At Mach 1, the airplane "breaks the sound barrier"
- Beyond Mach 1, airplane is now in front of its own sound wave

Ch8-101

Sonic Booms

- Compressions pile upon one another rather than being separated by rarefactions
- A very large compression is created with considerable energy
- Called a <u>sonic boom</u>
- Energy sufficient to break windows

Ch8-102

Section II
Practice Problems

CHAPTER 1

Practice Problems

Name:_____ Date:_____

1. You have two pendulums of different lengths. Why will the shorter pendulum vibrate with a higher frequency than the longer one?

2. Why does an object traveling with a velocity of 80 kph have greater momentum than the same object traveling with a velocity of 50 kph?

3. Describe the relation between the direction of vibration of the medium and the direction of wave propagation for a transverse wave.

4. Express 1.5 pascals (**Pa**) in equivalent newtons per square meter (**N/m^2**) and equivalent dynes per square centimeter (**dyne/cm^2**).

5. What derived physical quantity defines the time-rate change in displacement?

6. What derived physical quantity defines the time-rate change in velocity?

7. List the three fundamental physical quantities and the unit of measure for each in the MKS system.

8. What acts as the restoring force in a vibrating spring-mass system?

9. Describe how the magnitudes of potential energy and kinetic energy vary with the magnitude of displacement (x) of a mass from equilibrium during vibratory motion.

10. Why can you ordinarily see a flash of lightning before you hear the crash of thunder?

11. The frequency of a sound wave in air is 100 Hz. If the same sound wave travels through a water medium, what will be the frequency of vibration?

CHAPTER 2

Practice Problems

Name:_____   Date:_____

■ SET 1

1. If rms = $\dfrac{A}{\sqrt{2}}$, A must =

2. If A = rms (1.414), rms must =

3. Given rms, write the equation for peak-to-peak.

4. Solve for rms sound pressure for each of the following values of peak sound pressure.

   a.   1.0   b.   1.5   c.   0.6   d.   3.8

   _____   _____   _____   _____

5. Solve for peak-to-peak sound pressure for each of the following values of rms sound pressure.

   a. 0.707   b.   1.0   c.   3.5

   _____   _____   _____

6. Solve for rms sound pressure that corresponds to each of the following peak-to-peak values.

   a.   1.0   b. 1.414   c.   10   d.   2.0   e.   18   f.   x

   _____   _____   _____   _____   _____   _____

7. Given a sinusoid with a maximum amplitude of 5 volts (where voltage is an electrical analog to acoustic pressure), solve for:

   a. rms =   _____   b. P-P =   _____

   c. mean square =   _____   d. FW_{avg} =   _____

   e. HW_{avg} =   _____   f. A =   _____

8. For each 10-fold increase in maximum amplitude, rms increases by a factor of:
   _____

9. For each 2-fold increase in maximum amplitude, the full-wave rectified average increases by a factor of: _____

10. If rms increases by a factor of two,

    a. mean square increases by a factor of: _____

    b. the full-wave rectified average increases by a factor of: _____

11. If rms voltage were increased from 10 volts to 100 volts, mean square voltage would increase by a factor of: _____

12. Under what condition will the numerical value of rms equal the numerical value of mean square?

13. If $FW_{avg} = \frac{2A}{\pi}$, then HW_{avg} = _____

14. If $HW_{avg} = 1.3$, FW_{avg} = _____

15. If rms = 1.5 V, mean square = _____

16. If rms increases by a factor of N, mean square increases by a factor of: _____

■ SET 2

1. If the period of a sinusoid is 150 ms, f = _____

2. If 1.5 cycles are completed within 5 ms, f = _____

3. Calculate f, in Hz, for each period:

    a.   0.002 s   b.   3 ms   c. 1,000 μs

    _____   _____   _____

4. Calculate T, in ms, for each frequency:

    a.   400 Hz   b. 800 Hz   c.   100 Hz   d. 500 Hz   e. 8000 Hz

    _____   _____ _____   _____ _____

5. Calculate f, in kHz, for each of the following:

    a.   100 Hz   b. 0.002 s   c.   1 MHz   d.   5 ms

    _____   _____ _____   _____

6. Draw a sinusoidal pressure function (instantaneous pressure) where f = 1000 Hz and rms sound pressure = 1.414 Pa. Label both coordinates.

7. Draw a function that shows the distribution of rms sound pressure as a function of time for a sinusoid with a frequency of 500 Hz and a maximum sound pressure of 0.707 Pa.

■ SET 3

1. Describe the relation between **particle displacement** (**x**) and **particle velocity** (**c**) during simple harmonic motion.

2. Describe the relation between **period** and **angular velocity**.

3. Describe the proportional relations between the **frequency** of a vibrating string and the **mass**, **length**, and **tension** of the string.

4. Describe the proportional relations between the **period** of a vibrating string and the **mass**, **length**, and **tension** of the string.

5. Sine wave **A** has a **frequency** of 100 Hz and a **starting phase** of 0°. Sine wave **B** has a **frequency** of 110 Hz and a **starting phase** of 90°. Describe the phasic relation between the two waves during the course of one period of vibration for sine wave **A**.

6. Describe the proportional relations between the **natural frequency** of a freely vibrating system and the **mass**, **stiffness**, and **compliance** of the system.

7. What happens to the **resistance** of a spring-mass system as **frequency** of vibration increases?

■ SET 4

1. Table 2–1 of the textbook listed the sines of selected angles from 0° through 360° at 11.25° intervals. In Figure 2–9 of the textbook, **sin** θ was then plotted as a function of θ in degrees. Assume you have a wave with a **maximum amplitude (A)** of 2 **Pa**. Calculate the **instantaneous pressures (p)** for each of the angles listed below for the first half of one cycle (three decimal places).

θ	p	θ	p
0.00	_____		
11.25	_____	101.25	_____
22.50	_____	112.50	_____
33.75	_____	123.75	_____
45.00	_____	135.00	_____
56.25	_____	146.25	_____
67.50	_____	157.50	_____
78.75	_____	168.75	_____
90.00	_____	180.00	_____

2. For the same sine wave in #1 ($p_{max} = 2$ **Pa**), how would the results differ if you were to continue the computations at $11.25°$ intervals for the second half of the cycle?

3. For the same sine wave in #1, calculate each of the following in **Pa** (two decimal places).

a. rms = _____

b. mean square = _____

c. HW_{avg} = _____

d. FW_{avg} = _____

4. Suppose $R = 600$ Ω, $X_m = 500$ Ω, and $X_c = 500$ Ω.

a. What is the value of **Z** in ohms? _____

b. Is the system in resonance? _____

c. If X_c were increased to 600 Ω, would $Z = R$? _____

Practice Problems

Name:_____   Date:_____

■ SET 1

1. Express the following values in scientific notation.

   a.   6875   b.   0.0064   c.   109.6

   _____   _____   _____

2. What is the base of 8^2? _____

3. Solve each of the following.

   a. 7^3 b. 0.2^4 c. $10^{2.2} \times 10^{1.8}$

   _____   _____   _____

   d. $2^5 \times 2^{-2}$ e. $2^2 + 2^2$ f. $(5 \times 10^3) \times (2 \times 10^2)$

   _____   _____   _____

   g. $(xyz)^0$ h. 5.764^1 i. $\left(\frac{1.6}{5.2}\right)^0$

   _____   _____   _____

   j. $(10^2)^3$ k. $(3^2)^2$ l. $(2^{2.5})^2$

   _____   _____   _____

m. $(4^2)^{1/2}$ n. $3^{4/2}$ o. 2^{-2}

_____   _____   _____

p. 10^{-3}

_____

■ SET 2

1. Solve the following.

a. $\log_3 27$ b. $\log_4 16$ c. $\log_4 16^2$ d. $\log_4 16^{-2}$

_____   _____   _____   _____

e. $\log_{10} 10$ f. $\log_2 2$ g. $\log_{67} 67$ h. $\log_e e$

_____   _____   _____   _____

i. $\log_{10} 10^2$ j. $\log_{10} 100$ k. $\log_2 4$ l. $\log_3 9$

_____   _____   _____   _____

m. $\log_{12} 144$ n. $\log_e e^2$ o. $\log_{4.4} 4.4^{16}$ p. $\log_{10}$

_____   _____   _____   _____

q. $\log_{10} (3+4+1+2)$

_____

2. Assume a base of 10 for the following.

a. $\log 54$ b. $\log 3.6$ c. $\log 0.4$

_____   _____   _____

d.   antilog 0.3010   e. antilog 1.5315   f. antilog 6.7202

_____   _____   _____

Practice Problems

Name:_____   Date:_____

Recall the two-step procedure for solving decibel problems: (1) Select the proper equation, and (2) form a ratio and solve the problem.

It will always be useful to inspect a problem to see if it involves powers of 2 (3 dB for intensity; 6 dB for pressure) or powers of 10 (10 dB for intensity; 20 dB for pressure). Even though some problems cannot be solved that way, you will be able to estimate the answers in many cases by using powers of 2 and powers of 10 to set upper and lower limits that bracket the correct answers. Try to solve as many problems as possible using powers of 2 and powers of 10 (to facilitate this, solve problems in order from a to z), and then use your calculator to check your computations.

■ SET 1

Convert each of the following intensity ratios to decibels.

a.	1:1	b.	10:1	c.	100:1	d.	1,000:1	e.	10^3:1
___		___		___		___		___	

f.	2:1	g.	3:1	h.	4:1	i.	5:1	j.	6:1
___		___		___		___		___	

k.	7:1	l.	8:1	m.	9:1	n.	1:2	o.	1:3
___		___		___		___		___	

p.	1:4	q.	1:5	r.	1:6	s.	1:7	t.	1:8
___		___		___		___		___	

u.   1:9   v.   1:10   w.   1:100   x.   1:1,000   y.   .001:1

_____   _____   _____   _____   _____

z. 10^{-3}:1   aa.   20:1   bb.   200:1   cc.   40:1   dd.   400:1

_____   _____   _____   _____   _____

ee.   60:1   ff.   600:1   gg. (2.45×10^{0}):1

_____   _____   _____

hh. (2.45×10^{1}):1   ii. $\dfrac{(2.45 \times 10^{1})}{10^{-12}}$:1   jj. $\dfrac{(2.45 \times 10^{-8})}{10^{-16}}$:1

_____   _____   _____

■ SET 2

Convert each of the following decibels to intensity ratios.

a.   0   b.   10   c.   20   d.   30

_____   _____   _____   _____

e.   40   f.   70   g.   3   h.   6

_____   _____   _____   _____

i.   9   j.   12   k.   23   l.   29

_____   _____   _____   _____

m.   46   n.   56   o.   76   p.   −10

_____   _____   _____   _____

q.   −20   r.   −30   s.   −23   t.   −36

_____   _____   _____   _____

u.   17   v.   62   w.   91   x.   5.4

_____   _____   _____   _____

y.   12.6

_____

■ SET 3

Calculate dB IL re: 10^{-12} watt/m^2 for each of the following values of sound intensity (I_x).

a. 10^{-12} b. 10^{-11} c. 10^{-10} d. 10^{-9}

_____ _____ _____ _____

e. 10^{-8} f. 2×10^{-8} g. 4×10^{-8} h. 8×10^{-8}

_____ _____ _____ _____

i. 1×10^{-3} j. 4×10^{-3} k. 1×10^{-2} l. 2×10^{-2}

_____ _____ _____ _____

m. 0.5×10^{-2} n. 0.5×10^{-5} o. 0.5×10^{-12} p. 0.25×10^{-12}

_____ _____ _____ _____

q. 1.4×10^{-4} r. 2.8×10^{-4} s. 1.65×10^{-6} t. 3×10^{-6}

_____ _____ _____ _____

■ SET 4

Calculate sound intensity (I_x) in watt/m^2 for each of the following values of dB IL re: 10^{-12} watt/m^2.

a. 0 b. 10 c. 20 d. 30

_____ _____ _____ _____

e. 40 f. 60 g. 13 h. 23

_____ _____ _____ _____

i. 36 j. 49 k. -10 l. -20

_____ _____ _____ _____

m. -3 n. -6 o. -13 p. -23

_____ _____ _____ _____

q.   −26   r.   41   s.   62   t.   73

_____   _____   _____   _____

u.   87   v.   16.8   w.   24.2   x.   38

_____   _____   _____   _____

y.   47

_____

■ SET 5

Convert each of the following pressure ratios to decibels.

a.   1:1   b.   10:1   c.   100:1   d.   1,000:1   e. 10^3:1

_____   _____   _____   _____   _____

f.   2:1   g.   3:1   h.   4:1   i.   5:1   j.   6:1

_____   _____   _____   _____   _____

k.   7:1   l.   8:1   m.   9:1   n.   1:2   o.   1:3

_____   _____   _____   _____   _____

p.   1:4   q.   1:5   r.   1:6   s.   1:7   t.   1:8

_____   _____   _____   _____   _____

u.   1:9   v.   1:10   w.   1:100   x.   1:1,000   y.   0.001:1

_____   _____   _____   _____   _____

z. 10^{-3}:1   aa.   20:1   bb.   200:1   cc.   40:1   dd.   400:1

_____   _____   _____   _____   _____

ee.   60:1   ff.   600:1   gg. 10^{-4}:1   hh. 10^{-5}:1   ii. 10^{-2}:1

_____   _____   _____   _____   _____

jj. 10^{-1}:1   kk. 10^{0}:1   ll. $\dfrac{10^{-4}}{10^{-4}}$ mm. $\dfrac{10^{-3}}{10^{-4}}$ nn. $\dfrac{(2\times10^{-4})}{(2\times10^{-4})}$

_____   _____   _____   _____   _____

oo. $\dfrac{(4\times10^{-4})}{(2\times10^{-4})}$ pp. $\dfrac{10^{-4}}{(2\times10^{-4})}$

_____   _____

■ SET 6

Convert each of the following decibels to pressure ratios.

a.   0   b.   20   c.   40   d.   60

_____   _____   _____   _____

e.   80   f.   100   g.   6   h.   12

_____   _____   _____   _____

i.   18   j.   24   k.   −6   l.   −12

_____   _____   _____   _____

m.   26   n.   46   o.   72   p.   −20

_____   _____   _____   _____

q.   −40   r.   10   s.   30   t.   50

_____   _____   _____   _____

u.   44   v.   17   w.   62   x.   5.5

_____   _____   _____   _____

■ SET 7

Calculate dB SPL re: 2×10^1 µPa for each of the following values of sound pressure (p_x) in µPa.

a. 2×10^1 b. 2×10^2 c. 2×10^3

_____   _____   _____

d. 2×10^4 e. 2×10^5 f. 10^5

_____   _____   _____

g. 4×10^1 h. 8×10^1 i. 8×10^4

_____   _____   _____

j. 2×10^0 k. 4×10^0 l. 4×10^3

_____   _____   _____

m. 1.05×10^6 n. 1×10^5 o. 0.5×10^5

_____   _____   _____

p. 4×10^5 q. 4.25×10^5 r. 8.5×10^5

_____   _____   _____

■ SET 8

Calculate sound pressure (p_x) in µPa for each of the following values of dB SPL re: 2×10^1 µPa.

a.   0   b.   6   c.   12   d. -6

_____   _____   _____   _____

e.   20   f.   40   g.   60   h.   3

_____   _____   _____   _____

i.   9   j.   10   k.   30   l.   50

_____   _____   _____   _____

m.   43   n.   46   o.   36   p.   34

_____   _____   _____   _____

q.   72   r.   16.8   s. -7 t. -8

_____   _____   _____   _____

■ SET 9

Calculate dB SPL re: 2×10^{-4} dyne/cm^2 for each of the following values of sound pressure (p_x) in dyne/cm^2.

a.   0.0002   b.   0.0004   c. 8×10^{-4} d. 2×10^{-4}

_____   _____   _____   _____

e. 4×10^{-4} f.   0.002   g. 2×10^{-3} h. 4×10^{-2}

_____   _____   _____   _____

i. 1×10^{-5} j. 2×10^{0}

_____   _____

■ SET 10

Calculate the total intensity in watt/m^2 that results from combining the following intensities from uncorrelated sources.

a. $10^{-8} + 10^{-8}$ b. $10^{-6} + 10^{-6}$

_____   _____

c. $(2 \times 10^{-6}) + 10^{-6}$ d. $(2 \times 10^{-6}) + (5 \times 10^{-6})$

_____   _____

e. $(2 \times 10^{-6}) + (5 \times 10^{-6}) + (2 \times 10^{-6})$ f. $(2 \times 10^{-6}) + (3 \times 10^{-5})$

_____   _____

■ SET 11

Calculate the intensity level re: 10^{-12} watt/m^2 that results from combining the intensities in Set 10.

a. _____   b. _____   c. _____

d. _____   e. _____   f. _____

■ SET 12

Calculate the sound pressure level that results from combining the following uncorrelated sound sources whose levels are given in dB SPL.

a.   20 + 20   b.   30 + 30   c.   46.2 + 46.2

_____   _____   _____

d.   20 + 20 + 20   e.   30 + 30 + 30   f. 46.2 + 46.2 + 46.2

_____   _____   _____

g.   60 + 70   h.   60 + 66   i.   60 + 70 + 80

_____   _____   _____

Practice Problems

Name:_____   Date:_____

1. One of the complex waves that was described in this chapter has the following characteristics: The fundamental frequency (f_0) is 125 Hz, and energy is present at odd and even integer multiples of f_0. The amplitude of the 4th harmonic is -6 dB relative to the amplitude of the 2nd harmonic and -12 dB relative to the amplitude of f_0. Name the complex wave and explain the reasons for your choice.

2. A sawtooth wave has a fundamental frequency (f_0) of 123 Hz and a starting phase of $90°$. The relative amplitude of the 5th harmonic is -14 dB re: the amplitude of f_0. What is the relative amplitude of the 10th harmonic?

3. Describe the important similarities and differences between a square wave and a triangular wave.

4. A complex, periodic waveform with energy at odd and even harmonics has a fundamental period of 5 ms. What is the frequency of the 6th harmonic?

5. If signal level is 70 dB SPL and noise level is 79 dB SPL, what is the signal-to-noise ratio in dB?

6. The lowest note on a tuned piano, A_1, has a frequency of 27.5 Hz. What is the frequency of A_6? Show your work.

7. If signal intensity is 10^{-5} watt/m^2 and noise intensity is 8×10^{-5} watt/m^2, what is the S/N ratio *in dB*? Show your work.

8. The waveform of white, or Gaussian, noise is aperiodic with equal energy in any frequency band 1 Hz wide (from $\mathbf{f} - 0.5$ Hz to $\mathbf{f} + 0.5$ Hz). Thus, white noise has the same amount of energy in every frequency band that is 1 Hz wide regardless of the value of $\mathbf{f}$. Suppose that the sound pressure level in any *one* band 1 Hz wide is 60 dB SPL, and further suppose that a particular white noise has 10,000 bands of energy, each of which is 1 Hz wide. Can you calculate the sound pressure level for the total noise, that is, for all 10,000 bands together?

9. A pulse train has a **pulse repetition frequency** of 200 Hz and a **pulse duration (P_d)** of 3 ms.

   a. What proportion of each period is occupied by each pulse? _____

   b. List the frequencies of the first five harmonics.

   _____ _____ _____ _____ _____

   c. List the frequencies in Hz of the lowest three nulls in the amplitude spectrum (no decimals).

   _____ _____ _____

   d. If the **pulse train** were replaced by a **single pulse** with $P_d = 3$ ms, list the frequencies in Hz of the lowest three nulls in the amplitude spectrum (no decimals).

   _____ _____ _____

CHAPTER 6

Practice Problems

Name:_____   Date:_____

■ SET 1

For each of the problems in this set, assume that you are dealing with a white noise that has the following characteristics:

Bandwidth $(\Delta f) = 10,000$ Hz
Over-all SPL = 90 dB re: 20 µPa

1. $L_{ps} =$ _____

2. Calculate the SPL at the output of each of the following filters.

a. Band-pass filter: Δf =   200 Hz; f_c = 400 Hz _____

b. Band-pass filter: Δf =   400 Hz; f_c = 400 Hz _____

c. Band-pass filter: Δf = 1000 Hz   _____

d. Low-pass filter: f_U = 1000 Hz   _____

e. High-pass filter: f_L = 9000 Hz   _____

f. 1-octave filter: f_c = 1000 Hz   _____

g. 1-octave filter: f_c =   500 Hz   _____

■ SET 2

1. When you analyze a white noise with a constant percentage bandwidth filter at several different values of f_c, the SPL at the output of the filter increases at a rate of _____ dB/octave or _____ dB/decade.

2. If L_{ps} = 40 dB SPL

    a. What is the value of the *sound pressure* in a band 1 Hz wide?   _____

    b. What is the value of the *sound pressure* in a band 10,000 Hz wide?   _____

■ SET 3

For each of the problems in this set, assume that you are dealing with a white noise that has the following characteristics:
        Bandwidth (Δf) = 5000 Hz
        Over-all SPL = 80 dB re: 20 µPa

1. L_{ps} = _____

2. Calculate the SPL at the output of each of the following filters.

    a. Band-pass filter: Δf = 200 Hz; f_c = 400 Hz _____

    b. Band-pass filter: Δf = 400 Hz; f_c = 400 Hz _____

    c. Band-pass filter: Δf = 1000 Hz   _____

    d. Low-pass filter: f_U = 1000 Hz   _____

    e. High-pass filter: f_L = 4000 Hz   _____

    f. 1-octave filter: f_c = 500 Hz   _____

3. A white noise is analyzed with a 1-octave filter at seven preferred center frequencies. The **octave-band level** for 125 Hz is 35 dB SPL re: 20 µPa.

    a. Calculate the following **octave-band levels**.

f_c	dB SPL
125	35
250	_____
500	_____
1000	_____
2000	_____
4000	_____
8000	_____

b. What is L_{ps} for the noise? _____

c. If you would have used a 1/3-octave filter instead of a 1-octave filter, what would be the **1/3 octave-band level** slope? _____

Practice Problems

Name:_____   Date:_____

1. An electrical sinusoid is directed to an amplifier such that the level of the input signal does *not* exceed the linear portion of the input-output function of the amplifier. When the *input* signal level is 200 μV, the output level is measured to be 3 mV. If the input level then were increased from 200 μV to 2 mV, what should the output level be? Explain your answer.

2. For the same amplifier, suppose you decide to *lower* the input level substantially in an effort to ensure a low percentage harmonic distortion. What will you sacrifice, and why?

3. When making a tape recording of a person reading a passage of text, you decide to *increase* the input gain so that most of the VU deflections occur at about +2 VU rather than, say, −5 VU in an effort to achieve an improved signal-to-noise ratio. What will you sacrifice, and why?

4. The upper limit of the linear portion of an input-output function is approximately 1 dyne/cm^2 (cgs system), which corresponds to 74 dB SPL re: 2×10^{-4} dyne/cm^2. Express the same outcome in dB SPL re: 20 µPa (MKS system).

5. An electrical sinusoid is directed to an amplifier with an input level sufficiently high that you exceed the linear portion of the input-output function of the amplifier. With the aid of an appropriate filter and voltmeter, you measure the output voltages for five harmonics of the distorted output signal: $V_1 = 400$ mV; $V_2 = 25$ mV; $V_3 = 40$ mV; $V_4 = 2$ mV; and $V_5 = 4$ mV. Calculate the *approximate* percentage harmonic distortion.

Practice Problems

Name:_____   Date:_____

1. The intensity of a sound in a free, unbounded medium is 95 dB SPL at a distance of 200 meters from the source. In accordance with the inverse square law, by how many dB will the SPL be decreased at a distance of 2,000 meters from the source? Show your work.

2. For Problem #1, what will be the SPL at a distance of 2,000 meters from the source? Show your work.

3. Explain why the following statement is correct: "According to the inverse square law, the intensity decreases by 6 dB for each doubling of the distance."

4. Describe the ways in which reflecting surfaces and absorbent materials in a medium should cause the inverse square law not to hold strictly.

5. In the discussion of standing waves and resonant frequency for a tube that is *open at one end and closed at the other end*, we stated that a **displacement node** (a point of no vibration) is always located at the closed end of the tube because the air is not free to move, and a **displacement antinode** (a point of maximum vibration) is always located at the open end where the air can move freely. We can also talk about a **pressure node** (a point of zero pressure) and a **pressure antinode** (a point of maximum pressure), because not only are the air particles moving (being displaced), but also sound pressure increases and decreases in the tube. Describe the relation between displacement and pressure nodes and antinodes.

6. The tube below is closed at both ends.
    1. Draw the **displacement pattern** for the second resonance, F_2.

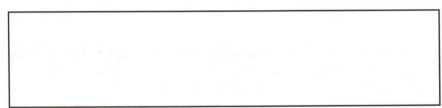

    2. If the speed of sound is 340 m/s and the length of the tube is 0.4 m, calculate F_2 (show your work):

        $F_2 =$ _____

7. A "fish locator," which more properly should be called a "depth finder," is a popular electronic device that can be used to measure water depth at a particular location on a body of water. The device emits a series of pulses from a transducer mounted on a boat just below the surface of the water, and the pulses travel to the bottom of the river or lake. How would you speculate that the device can reveal the water depth?

8. An empty classroom has the following dimensions: 10 m wide; 20 m long; and 3 m high. The floor is covered with heavy carpet and the walls and ceiling are constructed with plaster. For f = 500 Hz, α for the carpeting is 0.4 and α for the plaster is 0.1.

a. Calculate the total absorption, **A'**, for the room.

	Surface Dimensions	Surface Area (S)	α	A
Side wall 1	_____	_____	_____	_____
Side wall 2	_____	_____	_____	_____
End wall 1	_____	_____	_____	_____
End wall 2	_____	_____	_____	_____
Floor	_____	_____	_____	_____
Ceiling	_____	_____	_____	_____

A' = _____ .

b. Calculate T_{60} in ms (show your work): _____ .

c. Replace the plaster on the ceiling and one end wall with acoustical tile (α = 0.76):

A' = _____ , and

T_{60} = _____ .

Section III
Answers to
Practice Problems

Answers to Practice Problems

1. We learned from Equation 1.13 that the **period** of pendular vibration is *directly proportional* to the square root of the length of the pendulum. Because **frequency** and **period** are inversely proportional, it follows that **frequency** is *inversely proportional* to the square root of the length of the pendulum. Thus, the frequency of vibration of the shorter pendulum will be greater than the frequency of vibration of the longer pendulum.

2. Because it is the same object that is traveling at two different velocities, we should assume that **mass** is a constant. We learned from Equation 1.9 that **momentum** is equal to the product of **mass** and **velocity**. Therefore, momentum is *directly proportional* to the velocity. Thus, the greater the velocity, the greater the momentum.

3. The direction of vibration of the medium is *perpendicular* to the direction of wave propagation through the medium for a **transverse wave**. In contrast, for a **longitudinal wave**, the direction of particle movement of the medium is *parallel* to the direction of wave propagation.

4. We learned from Equation 1.7 that:

   $$1 \text{ Pa} = 1 \text{ N/m}^2 = 10 \text{ dynes/cm}^2.$$

   It follows, therefore, that:

   $$1.5 \text{ Pa} = 1.5 \text{ N/m}^2 = 15 \text{ dynes/cm}^2.$$

5. **Velocity**, which is the amount of displacement per unit time, or the ratio of the measure of displacement to the measure of time.

6. **Acceleration**, which is the time-rate change in **velocity**.

7. **Length** (meter), **mass** (kilogram), and **time** (second).

8. **Elasticity**. In contrast, **gravity** is the restoring force with pendular motion.

9. When **displacement** (x) is maximal, motion is momentarily halted, **potential energy** is greatest, and **kinetic energy** = 0. When $x = 0$ (as the mass passes through equilibrium), **potential energy** = 0, and **kinetic energy** is maximal.

10. The speed of light (299,792,458 m per s) is nearly 1 million times faster than the speed of sound (331 m per s at sea level with a temperature of 0° centigrade).

11. **100 Hz. Frequency** of vibration is dependent on properties of the source, which in this case is 100 Hz. The sound wave will be transmitted through the water with a greater **propagation speed** (about 4.3 times faster), but that is not relevant to answering the question.

Answers to Practice Problems

■ **SET 1**

1. rms $(\sqrt{2})$; or rms (1.414); or $\left(\dfrac{\text{rms}}{0.707}\right)$

2. $\dfrac{A}{1.414}$; or A (.707)

3. 2 (rms$\sqrt{2}$); or 2 (rms × 1.414); or $2\left(\dfrac{\text{rms}}{0.707}\right)$

4. a. 0.707   b. 1.06   c. 0.42   d. 2.69

5. a. 2   b. 2.828   c. 9.9

6. a. 0.35   b. 0.50   c. 3.5   d. 0.707   e. 6.36   f. 0.5x (.707)

7. a. 3.53   Given by 5 × 0.707

   b. 10   Given by 5 × 2

   c. 12.5   Given by $\dfrac{A^2}{2}$

   d. 3.18   Given by $\dfrac{2A}{\pi}$; or A (.636)

   e. 1.59   Given by $\dfrac{A}{\pi}$; or A (.318)

   f. 5   Given

8. 10

9. 2

10. a. 4   b. 2

11. 100

12. rms = 1   Because mean square = rms^2, and $1^2 = 1$

13. $\frac{A}{\pi}$

14. 2.6

15. 2.25 V^2

16. N^2

■ SET 2

1. 6.67 Hz

2. 300 Hz   Note that 1.5 cycles is to 5 ms as 1 cycle is to X ms. This is generally noted in the form 1.5 / 5 : 1 / X. The equation then is solved by cross-multiplication: 1.5X = 5 / 1; X = 3.33 ms. Therefore, if T = 3.33 ms, f = 1 / 3.33 = .3 kHz = 300 Hz.

3. a. 500   b. 333   c. 1000

4. a. 2.5   b. 1.25   c. 10   d. 2   e. 0.125

5. a. 0.1   b. 0.5   c. 1000   d. 0.2

6.

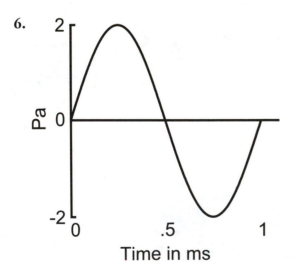

7.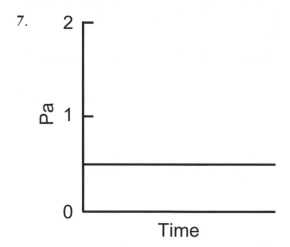

■ SET 3

1. **Particle velocity** *leads* **particle displacement** by 90°. For example, when particle displacement is 0°, particle velocity is 90°.

2. **Period** is *inversely proportional* to **frequency** ($T = 1/f$) and **frequency** is *directly proportional* to **angular velocity** ($\omega = 2\pi f$). Therefore, **period** must be *inversely proportional* to **angular velocity**.

3. **Frequency** is *inversely proportional* to twice the **length** of the string, *inversely proportional* to the square root of the string's **mass**, and *directly proportional* to the square root of the string's **tension**. See Equation 2.10.

4. Because **period** is *inversely proportional* to **frequency**, it follows that **period** is *directly proportional* to twice the **length**, *directly proportional* to the square root of the **mass**, and *inversely proportional* to the square root of the **tension**.

5. Because the two waves differ in frequency, the phasic relation between the two will vary from moment to moment; the difference of 90° in the two starting phases will *not* be preserved throughout the period.

6. The **natural frequency** of the system is *inversely proportional* to the square root of the **mass** and *directly proportional* to the square root of the **stiffness**. Because **compliance** is *inversely proportional* to **stiffness**, the **natural frequency** is *inversely proportional* to the square root of the **compliance**.

7. Nothing. **Resistance** is the energy-dissipating component of the **impedance** of the system and is *independent of frequency*. In contrast, **mass reactance** and **compliant reactance**, the energy-storage components of impedance, are frequency dependent: **mass reactance** is *directly proportional* to **frequency**, whereas **compliant reactance** is *inversely proportional* to **frequency**.

■ SET 4

1. p_{max} is 2 **Pa** and will be achieved at 90° where **sin** θ = 1.00. The sine of a given angle indicates the proportion (percentage if multiplied by 100) of p_{max} that is realized at that angle. Thus, to calculate the instantaneous value of **p** for a given angle, multiply the sine of that angle by p_{max} (2 **Pa** in this case).

θ	Pa	θ	Pa
0.00	0.000		
11.25	0.390	101.25	1.962
22.50	0.766	112.50	1.848
33.75	1.112	123.75	1.662
45.00	1.414	135.00	1.414
56.25	1.662	146.25	1.112
67.50	1.848	157.50	0.766
78.75	1.962	168.75	0.390
90.00	2.000	180.00	0.000

2. The values of **p** would be the same as in #1, but the sign would be negative (−). For example, if θ = 11.25°, **sin** θ = .195, and **p** = 0.390 **Pa** (−.195 × 2). Then if θ = 191.25° (180° + 11.25°), **sin** θ = −.195, and **p** = −0.390 **Pa** (−.195 × 2).

3. a. 1.414 Pa

   b. 1.999 Pa² (or 2.0 Pa²)

   c. 0.637 Pa

   d. 1.272 Pa

4. a. **500 Ω**. $Z = \sqrt{R^2 + (X_m - X_c)^2}$. Because $X_m = X_c$, **Z = R**.

   b. **Yes**. A system is in resonance when $X_m = X_c$.

   c. **No**. When $X_m \neq X_c$, **Z > R**. In this case, where **R** = 600 Ω, **Z** = 608 Ω.

Answers to Practice Problems

■ SET 1

1. a. 6.875×10^3 b. 6.4×10^{-3} c. 1.096×10^2

2.   8

3. a. 343; or 3.43×10^2 $(7 \times 7 \times 7)$
   b. 0.0016; or 1.6×10^{-3} $(.2 \times .2 \times .2 \times .2)$
   c. 10,000; or 10^4 $(10^{2.2 + 1.8} = 10^4)$
   d. 8; or 8×10^0 $(2^{5+(-2)} = 2^3)$
   e. 8; or 8×10^0 You are adding, not multiplying; Law 1 does not apply
   f. 10^6 $(10 \times 10^{3+2})$
   g. 1   Any base raised to the 0 power = 1
   h. 5.764   Any base raised to the 1st power = base
   i. 1   Same rule as for Problem 3-g; therefore, you need not divide 1.6 by 5.2

   j. 10^6 $(10^{2 \times 3})$
   k. 81; or 8.1×10^1 (3^4)
   l. 32; or 3.2×10^1 (2^5)
   m. 4 $(4^{2 \times 0.5} = 4^1 = 4)$
   n. 9 (3^2)
   o. 1/4; or 2.5×10^{-1} $(2^{-2} = 1 / 2^2 = 1/4)$
   p. 0.001 $(1 / 10^3)$

■ SET 2

1. a. 3   b. 2   c. 4   d. −4
   e. 1   f. 1   g. 1   h. 1
   i. 2   j. 2   k. 2   l. 2
   m. 2   n. 2   o. 16   p. −1
   q. 1

2. a. 1.7324   b. 0.5563   c. $\overline{1}.6021$; or −0.3979
   d. 2   e. 34   f. 5,250,000; or 5.25×10^6

Answers to Practice Problems

■ SET 1

Equation 4.4 should be used to convert the intensity ratios to decibels. In each of these problems, the reference is not specified, but the ratio I_x/I_r is known. For example, if the intensity ratio is 12:1,

$$N(dB) = 10 \log 12$$
$$= 10 \times 1.08$$
$$= 10.8 \text{ dB.}$$

a.	0	b.	10	c.	20	d.	30	e.	30
f.	3	g.	4.8	h.	6	i.	7	j.	7.8
k.	8.5	l.	9	m.	9.5	n.	−3	o.	−4.8
p.	−6	q.	−7	r.	−7.8	s.	−8.5	t.	−9
u.	−9.5	v.	−10	w.	−20	x.	−30	y.	−30
z.	−30	aa.	13	bb.	23	cc.	16	dd.	26
ee.	17.8	ff.	27.8	gg.	3.9				
hh.	13.9	ii.	133.9	jj.	83.9				

Notes

(a).   0 dB does not mean "silence." It means only that $I_x = I_r$ and, therefore, that the ratio $I_x/I_r = 1.0$ regardless of the absolute value of I_x.

(b,c,d).   You should note that each of these involves powers of 10, and each power of 10 corresponds to 10 dB. Thus, in 1-c the ratio is 100, which is a power of 10 twice (10^2). Because each power of 10 corresponds to 10 dB, the answer is given by 10 dB + 10 dB = 20 dB.

(f).   A power of 2, which is 3 dB.

(h).   Another power of 2. The ratio 4:1 corresponds to a power of 2 twice (2^2), and each power of 2 is 3 dB. Thus, 3 dB + 3 dB = 6 dB.

(i).   Can you see that the ratio 5:1 involves powers of 10 and powers of 2? The ratio 5:1 can be thought of as the ratio 10:1 (+10 dB) divided by the ratio 2:1 (−3 dB), which is 7 dB.

(1).   A power of 2 three times (2^3), which therefore involves 3 dB + 3 dB + 3 dB = 9 dB.

(n–z).   These are the inverse of the otherwise identical problems that were solved earlier in this set. Because the absolute value of $I_r > I_x$, the answer in decibels will be negative. Solution of such problems is simplified by recalling Log Law 4 (log 1/a = − log a). Thus, for example:

$$10 \log \frac{1}{2} = -10 \log 2 = -3 \text{ dB}.$$

(aa–dd).   By now you should quickly see that each involves a combination of powers of 10 (10 dB) and powers of 2 (3 dB). Thus, 400 consists of a power of 10 twice (+20 dB) and a power of 2 twice (+6 dB): $10 \times 10 \times 2 \times 2 = 400$, and the corresponding quantities in decibels are 10 dB + 10 dB + 3 dB + 3 dB = 26 dB.

(ee,ff).   These can only be approximated by powers of 2 and 10. To see how the approximation works, consider the ratio 600:1. You know that 400 ($10 \times 10 \times 2 \times 2$) is 26 dB and that 1,000 ($10 \times 10 \times 10$) is 30 dB. So, the answer for 600 must lie between 26 dB and 30 dB. If you think back to problem 1-i, you should be able to set the limits even closer. You solved that 5:1 is 7 dB (10/2). If 5:1 is 7 dB, 500 must be another 20 dB, for a total of 27 dB. Therefore, because 600 lies between 500 and 1,000, the answer must lie between 27 and 30. See if you can find a way, still using powers of 2 and 10, to lower the upper limit. (*Hint:* you should be able to set the upper limit to 29 dB.)

(gg,hh).   Solution of these problems is made easy by recalling two concepts from Chapter 3. First, both problems involve the log of a product. We learned from Log Law 1 that "log ab = log a + log b." Thus, with Problem 1-gg, we need only to add the logs of the two factors: $\log 2.45 + \log 10^0$. You will need a calculator or log table to determine the log of 2.45, but a second concept from Chapter 3 will allow you to determine the log of 10^0 without reference to a log table: "An exponent is a log, and a log is an exponent." Thus, the log of 10 raised to any power is the value of the power. Log $10^0 = 0$; log $10^1 = 1$; log $10^2 = 2$; . . . . ; log $10^n = n$.

(ii,jj).   These problems represent application of two laws of logarithms and one law of exponents. As a consequence, the problems can be solved in two ways. We will use 1-ii as an example. We can apply Log Law 1, where a = 2.45 and b = $(10^1 / 10^{-12})$. The log of 2.45 is determined from a calculator or log table, but there are two approaches available for determining the log of the ratio $10^1 / 10^{-12}$. With the first approach we apply Log Law 2: log a / b = log a − log b. Because we know that an exponent is a log, the log of that ratio is given by the difference between the exponents, $1 - (-12)$, which is 13. From Log Law 1, then, the log of the product is 0.4 + 13 = 13.4, which multiplied by 10 = 134 dB. With the second approach we apply Law 2 of exponents, which is a companion to Log Law 2: $X^a / X^b = X^{a-b}$. Therefore,

$$\frac{10^1}{10^{-12}} = 10^{13}$$

$$\log 10^{13} = 13$$
$$\text{and}$$
$$\text{dB} = 10 \,(0.4 + 13) = 134 \text{ dB}.$$

Why do both approaches give the same answer? With one we use Log Law 2. With the other we use the second law of exponents. *We get the same answer because a log is an exponent.*

■ SET 2

Equation 4.4 also should be used to convert each of the decibels to intensity ratios. Note that you are not solving for the absolute intensity, I_x, but just the ratio of the two intensities, I_x/I_r. For example, if dB = 5,

$$5 = 10 \log X$$
$$0.5 = \log X \qquad \text{(dividing both sides of the equation by 10)}$$
$$X = 3.16 \qquad \text{(the ratio of the unknown } I_x \text{ to the unknown } I_r\text{)}.$$

a.	10^0:1 (1:1)	b.	10^1	c.	10^2	d.	10^3
e.	10^4	f.	10^7	g.	2	h.	4
i.	8	j.	16	k.	2×10^2	l.	8×10^2
m.	4×10^4	n.	4×10^5	o.	4×10^7	p.	10^{-1}
q.	10^{-2}	r.	10^{-3}	s.	5×10^{-3}	t.	2.5×10^{-4}
u.	5×10^1	v.	1.58×10^6	w.	1.26×10^9	x.	3.47×10^0
y.	1.82×10^1						

Notes

(a–f).   Each of the decibel values is divisible evenly by 10, and each 10 dB of intensity corresponds to a power of 10. Thus, for these six problems, the solutions are a power of 10: the powers of 0, 1, 2, 3, 4, and 7, respectively. A second, but not independent, approach is to recall that, when you convert decibels to intensity ratios, the first step is to divide by 10. The result is a log, which in these cases is an integer of 0, 1, 2, 3, 4, and 7 followed by .0000. The integers are the characteristics, and they indicate the exponents in scientific notation. Thus, the results are 10^0, 10^1, 10^2, 10^3, 10^4, and 10^7.

(g–j).   Each of these is a value that is evenly divisible by 3, and each 3 dB corresponds to a power of 2. Thus, the answers are 2, 4, 8, and 16.

(k–o).   Each of these involves a combination of powers of 10 and powers of 2. For example, 2-k is 23 dB, and 23 dB consists of 10 + 10 + 3. Each 10 dB is a power of 10, and each 3 dB is a power of 2. Thus, the answer is $10 \times 10 \times 2 = 200 = 2 \times 10^2$.

(p–t).   Each of these involves either a power of 10 or a combination of powers of 10 and powers of 2. Because the decibel is negative, we know that *the exponent will be negative.* Thus, 10 dB corresponds to 10^1, whereas −10 dB corresponds to 10^{-1}.

(u).   Although you might not see it on first inspection, this problem also can be solved with powers of 10 and 2. Actually, 17 comprises 10 + 10 − 3. Thus, 17 dB would correspond to a tenfold increase in intensity twice, and a halving of intensity once: $(10 \times 10) / 2 = 50$. If the problem had involved 14 dB, could you have used the same approach? Yes. 14 = (10 + 10 − 3 − 3). Thus, 14 dB corresponds to: $(10 \times 10) / (2 \times 2) = 25$.

(v,w).   These, too, can be worked as combinations of powers of 10 and 2, but it might be quicker to solve them step-by-step with a log table or more quickly with your calculator rather than to spend time seeing if the powers of 10 and 2 rules apply. It is surprising, however, to see how many problems can be solved in that simple way without use of log tables or calculators. Consider 2-v. 62 dB = 10 + 10 + 10 + 10 + 10 + 3 + 3 + 3 + 3. So, we have a power of 10 five times (10^5) and a power of 2 four times (2^4). That corresponds to 16×10^5, which is 1.6×10^6 in scientific notation. Can you see how Problem 2-w can be approached in the same way? (*Hint:* You need to sum 10s and subtract 3s.)

(x,y).   There is no quick solution available for these, but you should be able to determine upper and lower limits to check to see if the answers you calculate are reasonable.

General Comment

We have emphasized that reasonably quick solutions to many problems can be realized by employing powers of 10 (10 dB) and powers of 2 (3 dB). Because the log of 2 = .30103, not 0.30000, you will sometimes experience a rounding error that might or might not be tolerable, depending on the accuracy that is required. Thus, 3 dB really corresponds to an intensity ratio of 1.9953:1 rather that 2:1, and that probably will not pose any difficulty most of the time. Look at problem 2-1, however. For 29 dB the answer was listed as 800:1, but the correct answer (two decimals) is 794.33:1. When greater accuracy is required, you should use the powers of 10 and powers of 2 shortcut only to estimate the answer and to aid you in determining if the answer you calculate is reasonable.

■ SET 3

Equation 4.4 also should be used for all of these problems. All problems in the set are conceptually identical to those in Set 1. The only difference is that in Set 1 you dealt only with a ratio of intensities (I_x/I_r) where the absolute values of I_x and I_r were unknown. In Set 3, both I_x and I_r are known. The first step, then, is to solve the ratio by reference to Law 2 of exponents ($X^a / X^b = X^{a-b}$), and the exponent in the result is the log of the ratio. For example,

$$
\begin{aligned}
dB &= 10 \log (10^{-7}/10^{-12}) \\
&= 10 \log 10^{(-7) - (-12)} \\
&= 10 \log 10^5 \\
&= 10 \times 5 \\
&= 50.
\end{aligned}
$$

a. 0	b. 10	c. 20	d. 30
e. 40	f. 43	g. 46	h. 49
i. 90	j. 96	k. 100	l. 103
m. 97	n. 67	o. −3	p. −6
q. 81.5	r. 84.5	s. 62.2	t. 64.8

Notes

(a–e).   Each involves a power of 10, and by now you should be able to solve these quickly. For example, in 3-c, 10^{-10} is two powers of 10 larger than the reference of 10^{-12}, each power of 10 corresponds to 10 dB, and the answer, therefore, is 20 dB.

(f–h).   These are combinations of powers of 10 and powers of 2.

(m).   This also is a combination of powers of 10 and powers of 2. Therefore, 10^{-2} involves 10 tenfold increases (100 dB). If 10^{-2} is 100 dB, then 0.5×10^{-2} (which is only half as great) must be 3 dB less, or 97 dB.

(q–r).   Problem 3-q cannot be solved by inspection. Having already solved 3-q, the answer to 3-r must be 3 dB greater than the answer to 3-q because 2.8×10^{-4} is twice as great as 1.4×10^{-4}.

■ SET 4

Equation 4.4 also should be used for these problems, which are conceptually identical to those in Set 2. The only difference is that in Set 2 you solved only for the intensity ratio (X), whereas in Set 4 you must carry the computation one step further to determine the actual value of I_x.

a.	10^{-12}	b.	10^{-11}	c.	10^{-10}	d.	10^{-9}
e.	10^{-8}	f.	10^{-6}	g.	2×10^{-11}	h.	2×10^{-10}
i.	4×10^{-9}	j.	8×10^{-8}	k.	1.00×10^{-13}	l.	1.00×10^{-14}
m.	0.50×10^{-12}	n.	2.50×10^{-13}	o.	0.50×10^{-13}	p.	0.50×10^{-14}
q.	0.25×10^{-14}	r.	1.26×10^{-8}	s.	1.58×10^{-6}	t.	2.00×10^{-5}
u.	5.00×10^{-4}	v.	4.79×10^{-11}	w.	2.63×10^{-10}	x.	6.30×10^{-9}
y.	5.00×10^{-8}						

Notes

(m).   If you followed the step-by-step procedures, you probably obtained 5×10^{-13} for your answer rather than 0.5×10^{-12} that is shown above, but the two answers are equivalent. The answer of 0.5×10^{-12} came from inspecting for powers of 2 and 10. We know that 0 dB corresponds to an intensity of 10^{-12}, so −3 dB must correspond to only half as much intensity, or 0.5×10^{-12}. The same explanation applies to Problems 4-n, o, p, and q.

(u–y).   Did you notice that you could solve these by inspection for powers of 10 and 2?

■ SET 5

Equation 4.7 should be used to convert the pressure ratios to decibels. Each of these problems is identical in concept to those in Set 1, and problems 5-a through 5-ff are identical numerically. The only difference is that now you are presented with pressure ratios rather than intensity ratios, and therefore the log of the pressure ratio is multiplied by 20 rather than by 10. Solution of the two sets of problems is otherwise identical.

Because the two sets of problems are virtually identical, except for the multiplier, there are no explanatory notes to accompany these problems. When in doubt, consult the notes for the corresponding problem in Set 1. As a general reminder, the vast majority of the problems can be solved by inspection for powers of 10 and powers of 2, where a power of 10 for pressure corresponds to 20 dB (20 log 10) and a power of 2 for pressure corresponds to 6 dB (20 log 2).

a.	0	b.	20	c.	40	d.	60	e.	60
f.	6	g.	9.5	h.	12	i.	14	j.	15.6
k.	16.9	l.	18	m.	19.1	n.	−6	o.	−9.5
p.	−12	q.	−14	r.	−15.6	s.	−16.9	t.	−18
u.	−19.1	v.	−20	w.	−40	x.	−60	y.	−60
z.	−60	aa.	26	bb.	46	cc.	32	dd.	52
ee.	35.6	ff.	55.6	gg.	−80	hh.	−100	ii.	−40
jj.	−20	kk.	0	ll.	0	mm.	20	nn.	0
oo.	6	pp.	−6						

■ SET 6

Equation 4.7 should be used to convert decibels to pressure ratios. The only difference in solutions of these problems from those encountered with Set 2 is that the first step is to divide by 20 rather than by 10 because the problems involve pressure rather than intensity.

a.	10^0 (1:1)	b.	10^1	c.	10^2	d.	10^3
e.	10^4	f.	10^5	g.	2	h.	4
i.	8	j.	16	k.	.5	l.	.25
m.	2×10^1	n.	2×10^2	o.	4×10^3	p.	10^{-1}
q.	10^{-2}	r.	3.16×10^0	s.	3.16×10^1	t.	3.16×10^2
u.	1.58×10^2	v.	7×10^0	w.	1.26×10^3	x.	1.88×10^0

■ SET 7

Equation 4.7 should be used for all of these problems, and all are identical in concept to the problems in Set 5. The only difference is that in Set 5 you dealt only with a pressure ratio (p_x / p_r) where the absolute values of p_x and p_r were not specified. In Set 7, both p_x and p_r are known. The first step, then, is to solve the ratio by use of the 2nd Law of exponents $(X^a / X^b = X^{a-b})$, and the exponent in the result is the characteristic in the log of the ratio. For example,

$$
\begin{aligned}
dB &= 20 \log (3 \times 10^3) / (2 \times 10^1) \\
&= 20 \log (1.5 \times 10^2) \\
&= 20 \times 2.18 \\
&= 43.6.
\end{aligned}
$$

a.	0	b.	20	c.	40
d.	60	e.	80	f.	74
g.	6	h.	12	i.	72
j.	−20	k.	−14	l.	46
m.	94.4	n.	74	o.	68
p.	86	q.	86.6	r.	92.6

Notes

Almost all of these problems can be solved by use of powers of 10 (20 dB) and powers of 2 (6 dB).

(a).   In this problem $p_x = p_r$, the ratio is therefore 1:1, the log of 1 is 0.0000, and the answer must be 0 dB.

(a-e).   As you proceed from 7-a through 7-e, you progressively increase by one power of 10 (10^1), which for pressure corresponds to increases of 20 dB. Thus, the answers are 0, 20, 40, 60, and 80 dB SPL.

(f-h).   Problem 7-f is one power of 2 (2^1) *less* than 7-e, which means that the sound pressure level for 7-f must be 6 dB less than the sound pressure level for 7-e. Similarly, you should see powers of 2 relations between 7-g and 7-a, between 7-h and 7-g, between 7-i and 7-d, and so on.

(m).   The value of p_x is only fractionally greater than 10^6. By using powers of 10 and 2 you should see that if p_x were 10^6, SPL = 94 dB (2×10^6 would equal 100 dB, so 1×10^6, which is half as much pressure, must be 6 dB less). If SPL = 94 dB when $p_x = 1 \times 10^6$, SPL must be only fractionally greater when $p_x = 1.05 \times 10^6$. Thus, the answer of 94.4 seems reasonable.

■ SET 8

Equation 4.7 also should be used for these problems, which are identical in concept to those in Set 6. The only difference is that in Set 6 you solved only for the pressure ratio (X), whereas in Set 8 you must carry the computation one step further to determine the actual value of p_x:

a.	2×10^1	b.	4×10^1	c.	8×10^1	d.	10^1
e.	2×10^2	f.	2×10^3	g.	2×10^4	h.	2.82×10^1
i.	5.64×10^1	j.	6.32×10^1	k.	6.32×10^2	l.	6.32×10^3
m.	2.82×10^3	n.	4×10^3	o.	1.26×10^3	p.	10^3
q.	8×10^4	r.	1.38×10^2	s.	8.93×10^0	t.	7.96×10^0

Notes

(a–g).   As with many decibel problems, laborious, step-by-step calculations can be avoided with problems 8-a through 8-g by inspecting to determine if powers of 2 (6 dB) or powers of 10 (20 dB) apply. In 8-a, 0 dB *always* means that $p_x = p_r$; therefore the answer must be 2×10^1. The answer to 8-b must be a power of 2 *greater* (6 dB) than the answer to 8-a, and therefore is 4×10^{-4}; 8-c is one power of 2 *greater* than 8-b; 8-d is one power of 2 *less* than 8-a; 8-e is one power of 10 (20 dB) *greater* than 8-a; 8-f is one power of 10 *greater* than 8-e; and 8-g is one power of 10 *greater* than 8-f.

(h,i). You need to calculate the answer to 8-h, but having done so, the answer to 8-i must be one power of 2 greater than 8-h because the difference between the two is 6 dB.

(j,k,l). You need to calculate the answer to 8-j, but having done so, you should see that 8-k and 8-l are powers of 10 relative to 8-j.

■ SET 9

Equation 4.7 should be used for all of these problems. The only difference between these and the problems in Set 7 is that pressure now is expressed in dynes/cm^2 (**cgs** system) rather than μPa, and the reference pressure (p_r) is 2×10^{-4} dyne/cm^2. For example,

$$dB = 20 \log \frac{(3 \times 10^{-4})}{(2 \times 10^{-4})}$$
$$= 20 \log 1.5$$
$$= 20 \times 0.18$$
$$= 3.6.$$

a.	0	b.	6	c.	12	d.	0
e.	6	f.	20	g.	20	h.	46
i.	−26	j.	80				

Notes

(a). The answer to 9-a must be 0 dB because $p_x = p_r$.

(b,c). The values of p_x in 9-b and 9-c are, respectively, one and two powers of 2 (each power of 2 corresponds to 6 dB) greater than the value of p_x in 9-a.

(d). 2×10^{-4} dyne/cm^2 is the same as 0.0002 dyne/cm^2 in 9-a.

(e–j). All of the remaining problems in Set 9 involve powers of 2 (6 dB) and/or powers of 10 (20 dB).

■ SET 10

You are asked to determine the *total intensity* in watts/m^2 rather than the *level* in decibels that corresponds to the total intensity. Therefore, you simply execute Steps 1 and 2 of the three-step procedure described in Set 12 that follows.

a.	2×10^{-8}	b.	2×10^{-6}
c.	3×10^{-6}	d.	7×10^{-6}
e.	9×10^{-6}	f.	3.2×10^{-5}

Notes

(f). The only difficulty, if any, that should be encountered is with 10-f. The key is that you must be certain that both intensities have the same exponent before you add. Thus, for example, $2 \times 10^{-6} = 0.2 \times 10^{-5}$, which when added to $3 \times 10^{-5} = 3.2 \times 10^{-5}$.

■ SET 11

The procedure used to solve these problems should have been sufficiently mastered that no explanation should be necessary.

a.   43   b.   63   c.   64.8
d.   68.5   e.   69.5   f.   75.1

■ SET 12

Even though the uncorrelated noise levels that are being combined are expressed in dB SPL, it is the energies, or powers, or intensities that should be added, not the pressures (See "Combining Sound Intensities from Independent Sources," Chapter 4). If the sources have equal intensity, you can use Equation 4.9:

$$dB_N = dB_i + 10 \log N.$$

For example, if five sources each produce a noise level of 72 dB,

$$dB_N = 72 + 10 \log 5$$
$$= 72 + 10 \,(0.7)$$
$$= 79.$$

If the source intensities are not equal, you must execute three calculations (*steps 1–3*).

1. Calculate the *intensity* in watt/m^2 for each source (Equation 4.4).

2. Add the intensities to determine the value of I_x to be used in the third step.

3. Calculate decibels with Equation 4.4 where $I_r = 10^{-12}$ watt/m^2. The result can be expressed as dB IL or dB SPL; they are equivalent.

For example, if two sources have noise levels of 80 dB SPL and 83 dB SPL:

Step 1:

$$80 = 10 \log \frac{I_x}{10^{-12}}; \text{ Therefore, } I_x = 10^{-4}.$$

$$83 = 10 \log \frac{I_x}{10^{-12}}; \text{ Therefore, } I_x = 2 \times 10^{-4}.$$

Step 2:

$$I_x + I_x = (1 \times 10^{-4}) + (2 \times 10^{-4})$$
$$= 3 \times 10^{-4}.$$

Step 3:

$$dB = 10 \log \frac{(3 \times 10^{-4})}{10^{-12}}$$

$$= 10 \log (3 \times 10^8)$$
$$= 10 \times 8.48$$
$$= 84.8 \ (dB \ IL \ or \ dB \ SPL).$$

a.	23	b.	33	c.	49.2
d.	24.8	e.	34.8	f.	51
g.	70.4	h.	67	i.	80.5

Notes

(a–f).   Problems 12-a through 12-f involve equal source intensities, which therefore permits you to solve the problems with Equation 4.9. Thus, for 12-a, the answer would be 20 + (10 log 2) = 23 dB. For 12-f, 46.2 + (10 log 3) = 51 dB.

(g,h,i).   For each of these problems you should use the three-step procedures described above. The solution for 12-i is shown below.

Step 1:

$$60 = 10 \log \frac{I_x}{10^{-12}}, = 10^{-6}.$$

$$70 = 10 \log \frac{I_x}{10^{-12}}, = 10^{-5}.$$

$$80 = 10 \log \frac{I_x}{10^{-12}}, = 10^{-4}.$$

Step 2: (Convert to common exponent of 10^{-4}.)

$$0.01 \times 10^{-4}$$
$$0.1 \ \times 10^{-4}$$
$$+ \ 1.0 \ \ \times 10^{-4}$$
$$= 1.11 \times 10^{-4}.$$

Step 3:

$$dB = 10 \log \frac{(1.11 \times 10^{-4})}{10^{-12}}$$

$$= 10 \log (1.11 \times 10^8)$$
$$= 10 \times 8.05$$
$$= 80.5$$

Answers to Practice Problems

1. **Sawtooth wave**. **Square waves** and **triangular waves** have energy at only *odd harmonics*. In addition, the wave in question has an envelope slope of -6 dB/octave, which also is consistent with a sawtooth wave.

2. **-20 dB**. The envelope slope of a **sawtooth wave** is -6 dB/octave. The level of the 5th harmonic is given as -14 dB, the 10th harmonic is one octave above the 5th harmonic, and therefore, the level of the 10th harmonic would be -20 dB. f_0 and **starting phase** are irrelevant.

3. Each has energy only at odd harmonics, but the envelope slopes are different: -6 dB/octave for a **square wave**, but -12 dB/octave for a **triangular wave**.

4. **1200 Hz**. If **T** $= 5$ ms, then $f_0 = 200$ Hz. The frequency of the 6th harmonic would be given by $6 \times 200 = 1200$ Hz.

5. **-9 dB S/N**. **dB S/N** is given by signal level in decibels *minus* noise level in decibels. Thus, $70 - 79 = -9$.

6. **880 Hz**. A_6 is five octaves above A_1. An octave is a doubling in frequency. Therefore, we multiply $27.5 \times 2^5 = 27.5 \times 32 = 880$.

7. **-9 dB**. Noise level is 8 times signal level, and $10 \log 8 = 9$ dB. Because noise level exceeds signal level, the **S/N ratio** would be -9 dB. Or, we could elect to use a longer procedure. With Equation 4.4 we calculate that **signal level** $= 70$ dB IL and that **noise level** $= 79$ dB IL. Therefore, **dB S/N** $= -9$ dB $(70 - 79 = -9)$.

8. With **white noise**, the starting phases of the 10,000 bands are in random array. Therefore, we can treat this as an instance of 10,000 *independent*, or *uncorrelated*, noise sources. Thus, with Equation 4.9 we calculate that:

$$\begin{aligned} dB_N &= dB_i + 10 \log N \\ &= 60 \text{ dB} + 10 \log 10{,}000 \\ &= 100 \text{ dB SPL}. \end{aligned}$$

9. a. **0.60 or 60%**. If the **pulse repetition frequency** = 200 Hz, T = 5 ms. P_d = 3 ms, which is 60% of 5 ms.

   b. The harmonics are *odd and even* integer multiples of the pulse repetition frequency: 200 Hz; 400 Hz; 600 Hz; 800 Hz; and 1000 Hz.

   c. Nulls are located at integer multiples of $1 / P_d$: 333 Hz; 667 Hz; and 1000 Hz.

   d. Nulls are located at integer multiples of $1 / P_d$, just as they were for the **pulse train**: 333 Hz; 667 Hz; and 1000 Hz.

Answers to Practice Problems

■ SET 1

1. 50 dB $\quad$ $L_{ps} = SPL_{wb} - 10 \log \Delta f = 90 - 10 \log 10,000.$

2. a. 73 dB $\quad$ $SPL_{wb} - 10 \log \dfrac{10,000}{200}$; or $L_{ps} + 10 \log 200$:

$\qquad\qquad$ Note: f_c is irrelevant; bandwidth was specified.

$\quad$ b. 76 dB $\quad$ f_c is still irrelevant.

$\quad$ c. 80 dB

$\quad$ d. 80 dB $\quad$ The key to solution of this problem is bandwidth.

$\quad$ e. 80 dB $\quad$ The bandwidth is the same as in 2-d.

$\quad$ f. 78.5 dB $\quad$ With a 1-octave filter you must calculate bandwidth: $\Delta f = f_c \times .707.$

$\quad$ g. 75.5 dB $\quad$ Either use the same procedure that you employed in 2-f or realize that this bandwidth is 1/2 as wide as that in 2-f, which means that the output in 2-g will be 3 dB less than that in 2-f.

■ SET 2

1. 3 dB/octave and 10 dB/decade

2. a. 2×10^3 $\quad$ $40 \text{ dB} = 20 \log \dfrac{p_x}{(2 \times 10^1)}$; $p_x = 2 \times 10^3.$

$\quad$ b. 2×10^5 $\quad$ If $L_{ps} = 40$ dB, then $SPL_{10,000} = 80.$ Now, solve for p_x.

■ SET 3

1. 43 dB $\quad$ $L_{ps} = SPL_{wb} - 10 \log \Delta f$

2. a. 66 $\quad$ b. 69 $\quad$ c. 73 $\quad$ d. 73 $\quad$ e. 73 $\quad$ f. 68.5

3. a. The preferred center frequencies for a 1-octave filter are spaced at octave intervals, and the **octave-band level** slope for white noise is +3 dB/octave. Therefore,

f_c	dB SPL	
125	35	(given)
250	38	
500	41	
1000	44	
2000	47	
4000	50	
8000	53	

   b. **15.5 dB SPL**. $L_{ps} = SPL_{wb} - 10 \log \Delta f_{wb}$. Your calculation of L_{ps} should be the same regardless of which of the seven outcomes in 3-a that you elected to use in the equation.

   c. **+3 dB/octave**. The slope will *not* be affected by your choice of constant percentage bandwidth filter.

Answers to Practice Problems

1. **30 mV**. Over the linear portion of the **input-output function**, the output level is *proportional* to the input level. The input signal increases by a factor of 10:1 (200 μV to 2 mV). Therefore, the output signal also should increase by a factor of 10:1, from 3 mV to 30 mV.

2. If the input level is reduced, the effective **signal-to-noise ratio** will be reduced because signal level will lie closer to the electrical noise floor of the system.

3. This is the reverse of the situation in the second problem. As you increase signal level to achieve a better **signal-to-noise ratio**, **percentage harmonic distortion** will increase because you now will be operating closer to, or on, the nonlinear portion of the input-output function.

4. **74 dB SPL**. A reference pressure of 2×10^{-4} dyne/cm^2 in the cgs metric system is equivalent to a reference pressure of 20 μPa in the MKS system.

5. **11.8%**. The problem is solved with Equation 7.2.

$$\text{percentage harmonic distortion} = \sqrt{\frac{V_2^2 + V_3^2 + V_4^2 + V_5^2}{V_1^2}} \times 100$$

$$= 11.8\%$$

Answers to Practice Problems

1. 20 dB
$$dB = -20 \log \frac{2,000}{200}$$
$$= -20 \log 10$$
$$= -20$$

(Equation 8.4)

2. 75 dB SPL
$$dB \ SPL = 95 - 20$$
$$= 75$$

3. The distance is doubled, which is a distance ratio of 2:1. Thus,
$$dB = -20 \log \frac{2}{1}$$
$$= -20 \times 0.3$$
$$= -6$$

4. With sound wave **reflection**, sound energy is retained in the medium. Therefore, attenuation over distance will be *less* than the amount predicted by the **inverse square law** where sound energy is not retained in the medium. With sound wave **absorption**, sound energy is absorbed by material in the medium and it is attenuated over distance. Thus, the total attenuation will be greater than would be predicted by the inverse square law.

5. Think back to Chapter 2 where we learned that pressure (and velocity) leads displacement by 90°; they are *not* in phase. Therefore, a **displacement node** will correspond to a **pressure antinode**, and a **displacement antinode** will correspond to a **pressure node**. Thus, at the *closed end* of the tube we have a **displacement node**, but a **pressure antinode**. At the *open end* of the tube we have a **displacement antinode**, but a **pressure node**. (See panel C of Figure 8–10.)

6. a.

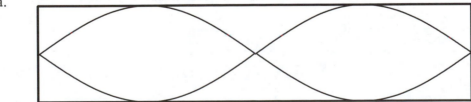

A **displacement node** must be located at each end of the tube. There should be two **displacement antinodes** located midway between adjacent nodes, one at 1/4 L and a second at 3/4 L.

b. **850 Hz.**

$$F_2 = \frac{2s}{2L}$$

$$= \frac{2 \times 340}{2 \times 0.4}$$

$$= 850 \text{ Hz.}$$

7. **Reflection** is the key. The pulses that travel from the instrument to the bottom of the river or lake are **incident pulses**. When they strike the bottom, they return to the instrument as **reflected pulses**. Because the reflected pulses travel with the same speed as the incident pulses, the instrument measures the total travel time and converts travel time to distance traveled. It also is possible to infer whether the bottom is hard (rocky) or soft (mucky). Hard surfaces will offer a larger impedance, and strong signals will be reflected back, whereas soft surfaces will offer a lesser impedance, more of the energy will be absorbed, and the reflected pulses will be weaker.

8. a.

	Surface Dimensions	Surface Area (S)	α	**A**
Side wall 1	20 × 3	60	0.10	6.0
Side wall 2	20 × 3	60	0.10	6.0
End wall 1	10 × 3	30	0.10	3.0
End wall 2	10 × 3	30	0.10	3.0
Floor	10 × 20	200	0.40	80.0
Ceiling	10 × 20	200	0.10	20.0

$$A' = 118.0.$$

b. **818 ms**

$$T_{60} = k \frac{V}{A'}$$

$$= .161 \frac{(20 \times 10 \times 3)}{118}$$

$$= .818 \text{ s}$$
$$= 818 \text{ ms}$$

c. **$A' = 269.8$ metric sabines; $T_{60} = 358$ ms.**
   A for the end wall increases from 3.0 to 22.8, **A** for the ceiling increases from 20.0 to 152.0, and **A'** increases from 118.0 to 269.8 **metric sabines**. Then,

$$T_{60} = .161 \frac{600}{269.8} = 358 \text{ ms.}$$